JUST HOW SMART IS PROZAC®?

It was hailed as a "Personality Pill";
making Prozac the hottest Psychiatric
drug in history.

JUST HOW SMART IS PROZAC®?

By
Makram Girgis, M.D., Ph.D.

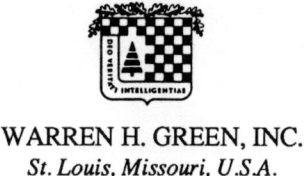

WARREN H. GREEN, INC.
St. Louis, Missouri, U.S.A.

Published by

WARREN H. GREEN, INC.
8356 Olive Boulevard
Saint Louis, Missouri, 63132 U.S.A.

© 1995 by WARREN H. GREEN, INC.

ISBN No. 0-87527-517-6

Printed in the United States of America

"What we are going to find out
about the brain is mind-boggling.
Every time a new drug is found,
another disease disappears, and makes
one very curious about what other
diseases have a biological basis."

-Dr. Paul Wender
Professor of Psychiatry

PREFACE

The rationale and structure of this book arose from the experience of preparing a "guide to patient's understanding and dealing with depressive disorder." This book is written by a doctor directed to general practitioners treating a crippling illness. Most depressed patients are brave. They are lost but not defeated. I hope that this book not only sustains hope throughout its pages, but it also backs it with a positive program for recovery.

I wish to thank all my patients for the understanding of their illnesses they have given me over the years. I have learned more about subtleties of emotional disorders from my patients, and in writing this book I made use of the way in which its can be explained to the layman.

Some recent articles and books talked about the "personality pill" in relation to Prozac. I sincerely believe Prozac is an excellent medication for treating severe depression. Actually the results in the majority of cases are remarkable. In seeking to distance myself from the claims made that "Prozac seemed to lend the introvert the social skills of a salesman", I have discussed fully in chapters II and XI this controversial issue. In these chapters, I have examined the interplay of forces that shape the individual's personality through the course of life,; promote, disrupt, or transform the personality across time. In chapter II, I outlined the theories of personality and how, in shaping personality, genetic and environmental influences do not act independently of one another, but are intertwined from the moment of birth.

Eli Lilly has also sought to distance itself from some media allegations that Prozac is a "wonder drug" which can improve "brain function, and increase intellectual capacity. The company has recently sent out a letter to all Doctors emphasizing that "these media allegations of 'wonder drug'" have no scientific basis and Lilly rejects them. Persistence of these media claims runs the risk of trivializing a serious disease and raising unrealistic expectations."

I have only prescribed Prozac when a diagnosis of major (and rarely moderate/ severe) depression is made. Its efficiency in such cases "has been firmly established in more than 10 million patients world-wide in 69 countries since it was first launched in 1986", however, it must be emphasized that the positive experiences are associated with patients recovery from depression so they are not necessarily specific to "Prozac" and could not be extrapolated to non-depressed people.

Modern psychiatrists have greater knowledge and farther horizons than their predecessors. The vantage point from which we survey the neuroscience is the product over many decades of great scientists. In assembling information from different sources and disciplines, the author may assume excessive liberty. Some meritorious contributions may have been regrettably overlooked.

The basic interest in this project began some 25 years ago when I started working at the Missouri Institute of Psychiatry at the St. Louis State Hospital Complex. I wish to thank many of my friends and senior colleagues who have given me a great deal of support and advice: Dr. George A. Ulett, who was formerly Director of the Missouri Division of Mental Health and the Missouri Institute of Psychiatry. He is presently Professor of Psychiatry at the Missouri Institute of Mental Health at St. Louis. Dr. Leopold Hofstatter who has been associated with the St. Louis State Hospital complex and the Missouri Institute of Mental Health for almost fifty years is presently Professor of Psychiatry at the Institute. I would like to express my gratitude to Dr. Danny Wedding, who is currently the new director of the Missouri Institute of Mental Health and Professor of Psychiatry, for the facilities that he has granted me during my recent visit to St. Louis so as to finalize the different chapters of my book. I am also grateful to his assistant, Vicki Eichhorn, and Alisa Mixon for clerical help, and to Mary Johnson, Nancy Casey and Susan Phiropoulos of the Institute library for their assistance.

Because of our mutual interest in the 'LIMBIC SYSTEM OF THE BRAIN', Dr. Paul D. MacLean and I have exchanged a great deal of correspondence and scientific communication for almost thirty years now. All this culminated in an invitation to visit his laboratories at the Section of Brain Evolution and Behavior, National Institute of Mental Health at Bethesda. I am grateful to him for a great deal of encouragement and inspiration.

Professor Leslie Kiloh, Professor Emeritus of Psychiatry, University of New South Wales and Dr. John Sydney Smith have given me a great deal of support and through their collaboration the First International Symposium on Limbic Epilepsy and the Dyscontrol Syndrome was held in Sydney in 1980.

I am indebted to my wife Claire for her patience and continued support and our children Marcelle, Marvet, Magda and Michael who, because of their interest in the bio-medical field, have always generated interesting and useful discussion. I am particularly grateful to my daughter Marvet for typing an important section of the manuscript. I am also grateful to Mrs. Julie Overall for typing many chapters of this book.

Lastly, but certainly not least, I must express my sincere gratitude to my publisher, Warren H. Green Inc., St. Louis, Missouri, who has so far published three of my books. The late Mr. Warren Green was not only a very good friend but, as a publisher, has given me a great deal of support and editorial advise. His wife Joyce, in following the excellent tradition of her husband, has been gracious enough to invite me to continue this happy and cordial relationship with Warren H. Green Inc.

St. Louis, Missouri   **Makram Girgis**

INTRODUCTION

Doctors have never been besieged to such an extent for any medication as is happening now with tranquilizers and antidepressants (particularly more recently with Prozac antidepressant).

Almost any phenomenon—bereavement, loss of job, difficulties involving a spouse or partner—can trigger off sensations of tension and anxiety. In a society where, increasingly, people are unwilling to make use of their own resources and will not tolerate disagreeable mood changes for long, the doctor is expected to provide chemical remedies.

General practitioners know they are in the front line of support for hundreds of thousands of people who have relatively minor disturbances because the stress of life they are leading is proving too much for them. They feel concerned that the whole burden of coping with this stress seems to have fallen on them. People know that doctors can mend broken limbs and they therefore go to the doctor to mend their damaged lives (the broken brain).

Doctors do not have a pill for every ill, a cure for every inconvenience of life. Sometimes, treating the symptoms is all doctors can do. They can't do what is hoped for and cure the cause. Some doctors may not realize how critical their initial response is to a new patient. An abrupt or dismissive reaction can be the final straw to a person who has found it impossible to talk to anyone else about their state of mind and regards the doctor as their only lifeline. Such patients need a considerate, human response.

Although my book is written for the general practitioner, I have great hopes that it will be of interest to the specialists as well. It is also hoped that the budding neuroscientists will benefit from the chapters discussing the neurotransmitter imbalance in mental disorders.

For the general practitioner, I have the chapter on cognitive behavior therapy, which will be of particular help in counseling the depressed patient (whether the patient is on medication or not).

Many millions of people throughout the world suffer from mild degrees of tension and depression. Only a few of them will ever see a psychiatrist. Far too often we hear the expression, "you must learn to live with it". This is not good enough.

Patients who are depressed or tense are eager to treat their general practitioner as counselor, adviser and trusted confident. However, many patients say their general practitioner doesn't listen to them; not easily approached about emotional problems as he or she would about hypertension or diabetes. Instead, he or she relies mainly on prescribing drugs for treating emotional problems.

Most doctors, however, even if they are interested in the counseling side, would say that they simply do not have the time to talk to patients at length. Stressed patients usually find their problems difficult to talk about quickly and cannot present all the facts neatly in ten minutes. Finding the cause of anxiety or depression can be a very lengthy business, particularly if the general practitioner is unskilled at it and it is disconcerting for the patient if the consultation is ended abruptly.

Even doctors who are willing to listen find that sometimes their patients are reluctant to tell them the real reason for their depression—or else have submerged their feelings so deeply that they are unaware of why they feel so low. Under Chapter VI (MASKED DEPRESSION), I have discussed fully this issue. Many patients also feel uncomfortable talking about psychological emotional problems in front of a highly qualified middle-class professional, who has only five minutes or so to spare them.

The patients are often in a bad mental state and they may often cloak it by complaining of physical ailments. A perceptive doctor, however, will see through the respectable medical symptoms and spot the warning sign of stress building up that the patient may not be aware of. Also, some patients want to know what sort of doctor they've got: cold, tough-minded, scientific or warm, friendly, understanding. So they try him out with a neutral symptom.

Doctors' attitudes to patients depends, to a certain extent, on their own personality; whether they are the "pull yourself together" type or prefer to adopt a bedside manner. In general though, doctors caught up in the general euphoria about the happiness pill have freely prescribed tranquilizers and antidepressants (such as PROZAC).

In Chapter VIII (COGNITIVE BEHAVIOR THERAPY), I have discussed at length the importance of this therapy whether the patient is on medications or not. A lot of patients are unhappy with their lives or their relationships or have goals which they haven't achieved. They may hide from their problems by asking for pills, but that doesn't solve anything. Unless they talk about what is upsetting them and get advice, they'll be on pills for years.

Cognitive behavioral assessment is based on simple principles and has clearly defined aims. The first, and perhaps central principle of cognitive behavioral assessment is that the ways in which an individual behaves are determined by immediate situations and the individual's interpretation of them. This therefore becomes the major focus of the assessment, with an emphasis on specific problems rather than global entities. This will be facilitated if there is a warm and trusting atmosphere, no risk of censure and if the therapist is empathic and clearly committed to helping the patient overcome current difficulties.

Doctors will sometimes prescribe medications in order to "please" the patient. After all, in the patient's eyes, the doctor is there to give tangible help. The very name of tranquilizers (and particularly more so PROZAC) beckons patients and doctors towards dreaming of a calm, serene existence.

Doctors also find themselves in a quandary when they are faced with patients in tears and under severe stress. Many are embarrassed or disconcerted by the emotion being shown and by the patients who show no signs of getting up and going. By handing them a prescription, the doctor can regain control of the situation and acceptably keep patients at arms' length.

Cognitive behavior therapy is now firmly established as the leading psychological treatment of patients suffering from a wide range of emotional disorders and numerous controlled trials have demonstrated its effectiveness.

Cognitive behavior therapy can be conceptualized as a type of problem-solving. Patients arrive with a number of problems, including depression itself. Depressive thinking prevents them from solving these. Tackling negative automatic thoughts is thus a means to an end not an end in itself. The goal of the therapy is to find solutions to the patient's problems, using cognitive-behavioral strategies, not merely to help the patient to think more "rationally". The immediate target is symptom-relief. At this stage an antidepressant such as Prozac is appropriate.

Psychiatry has not always been recognized as a biological science. Its assured status today owes much to the appreciation of the role of the limbic system of the brain in behavioral science and in fact arose pari passu with our understanding of that system which is concerned with memory and the control of emotional behavior. This issue is discussed fully in Chapter V (DISORDERS OF THE LIMBIC SYSTEM OF THE BRAIN). Research in this field may be regarded as the ultimate quest of the scientist and should lead man to a richer comprehension of himself, his fellow man and problems of society.

I believe firmly that science is a steady, logical accumulation of knowledge which will bring us even closer to the truth. We are currently approaching the end of a long period of relative tranquility in the health sciences. The signs of revolution are everywhere: within the health professions there has been a dramatic ascendancy of holistic medicine and humanistic psychology. Other factions have brought empirical disciplines such as acupuncture and Eastern meditations to the public's attention in search of "better mental health". In Chapter III, I discussed this issue and in particular "THE BIO-MEDICAL

REVOLUTION IN PSYCHIATRY."

We have still not achieved a definitive hypothesis for the neuro-chemical basis of most mental disorders. As research in psychopharmacology moves with increasing direction and sophistication in the level of neurotransmitters there are signs that we may be advancing in the right direction. It is possible that we may find the answers to the causes of affective disorders in the not too distant future.

Antidepressant drugs were introduced into clinical practice in the late 1950's. The bench-mark study for antidepressant drugs, which subsequently had considerable reverberations, was the multicenter trial of IMIPRAMINE. Investigation of and speculation about the role of biogenic amines (brain neurotransmitters) in the mediation of mood and in the psychopathology of affective disorders has occupied a great deal of attention in the past decade. In the early and mid-sixties it was hypothesized that clinical depression was associated with a functional deficiency of the neurotransmitters norepinephrine or serotonin at crucial reception sites in the brain, while mania would be associated with a function excess of these amines. Tricyclic antidepressants, such as Tryptanol, were used for a long time although the side effects somehow limited their use and efficiency.

More recently, in an attempt to manufacture antidepressants without the adverse effects of the tricyclics, many novel compounds have been introduced. In almost every case, it has been claimed that the drug is safer and better tolerated than previous ones and that it is especially suited to the elderly patient.

Although in some parts of the world the number of Prozac prescriptions is only a fraction of those written for the Tricyclic drugs, the most commonly prescribed antidepressants—the extraordinary hype that has surrounded Prozac in the U.S. has filtered throughout the world. It is not uncommon for patients to ask specifically for Prozac which is unprecedented for an antidepressant.

Prozac, which became available in the U.S. in 1987, is the brand name of the chemical Fluoxetine. Since its introduction in the U.S. more than six million Americans have used it; more than ten million people have used it worldwide, making it the world's number one prescribed antidepressant. What sets Prozac apart from other antidepressants is that it is the first drug to come on the market without apparent side effects. As mentioned above, a deficiency in the brain neurotransmitter, serotonin may cause depression. Prozac prevents nerve cells from taking up and destroying serotonin, leaving more in the neurotransmission system. The effects are dramatic.

I must admit that when I first started prescribing Prozac some two years ago, some of my patients asked or at least inquired about it. When a middle aged lady said to me: "After seven weeks Prozac has literally saved my life," I was surprised. This patient was a very cynical person and never believed that any treatment would ever help her. Not surprisingly so, as for twenty years she was subjected to every therapeutic modality, including the notorious "deep sleep therapy." She was referred to me two years ago because it was thought that the CT brain scan showed some indication of minor atrophic changes in the temporal lobe.

Several investigators did a double-blind clinical trial to evaluate the clinical efficiency and safety of Fluoxetine compared with imipramine in the treatment of major depression. The mean score of all depression rating scales showed that the drugs had comparable efficiency—The side effects profile of imipramine were anticholinergic and also excessive sedation—Thus the compliance difficult.

However, as will be reported in more detail in Chapter XI (PROZAC: BETTER FUTURE), the great majority of the patients who were suffering from major depression responded dramatically to Prozac. The results were in some patients just miraculous, particularly when compared to the tricyclic results. The majority of my 150 patients were on tricyclic at one stage. They either did not respond well or had to stop taking tricyclics because of frequent side effects.

Although it is a bit difficult to remember all the reasons why I was slow in accepting Prozac at the outset, a couple of issues could have influenced my judgment. For almost thirty years now I have been researching the role of the "cholinergic" limbic system of the brain (rather than the aminergic system) in trying to find the cause of depression, dementia and epileptic disorders. The term "cholinergic" pertains to the other major neurotransmitter in the brain called acetycholine (in contrast to the biogenic amines mentioned above—norepinephrine and serotonin).

In an article entitled "critique of a single neurotransmitter theory of depression," I explained that my investigations indicate that central cholinergic factors may play an important role in the causes of depression. The central anticholinergic action of tricyclic antidepressants has been sorely neglected, although it may play an important role in re-establishing the disturbed neurotransmitter imbalance in depressive illness. So far, the prime emphasis has been placed on the effect of these agents on the mono-aminergic system in depression.

The resulting prevalence of the cholinergic system and disequilibrium between stimulating and inhibiting neurotransmitters has failed to gain adequate attention. The available evidence of central anti-cholinergic action has so far been mainly inferential; their peripheral anti-cholinergic effect (dry mouth, blurred vision) seemed to indicate an equivalent central effect to be very likely. Not many scientists linked this possibility with the therapeutic effectiveness of the tricyclics.

However, because of the remarkable results of Prozac (which is linked to the competitor neurotransmitter—serotonin), I have recently been intrigued by this hypothesis of depression. A rational explanation for the mode of action of all antidepressant drugs cannot be offered through one unifying theory, but one that best fits the purpose of bringing together the action of many of these drugs involves their interactions with the dynamics of central monoamines.

I have found that with most of my patients, the results of Prozac in agitated depression were better when it was combined in the early stages with the "sedative" action of small doses of tricyclics which could very well be cholinergic. If the patient is unable to take tricyclics, then a mild tranquilizer at night will be most helpful for the first four weeks.

Prozac (Fluoxetine) is two hundred times more active in inhibiting (selectively) the uptake of serotonin than of norepinephrine—and it did not affect the histamine or acetylcholine—as in the case of some tricyclics. Fluoxetine was therefore hailed as a **clean drug**. Prozac is safer in the hands of potentially suicidal patients who might attempt to overdose on the drug. Because of the medical likelihood of effects on the heart, Prozac overdoses are relatively benign. Safety in overdose is a major advantage of Prozac over older antidepressants. No deaths occurred in patients receiving Fluoxetine at normal doses in clinical trials. Two deaths involving a Fluoxetine (plus another drug) overdose were reported during comparative clinical trials. Another 32 patients recovered without lasting harm from overdose, including one who reportedly took 3000mg of Fluoxetine; over 37 times the recommended maximum dose.

Fifteen percent of patients with depressive disorders commit suicide. The side effects associated with some tricyclics usually led to subtherapeutic dosing, premature discontinuation of therapy, or lack of patients' compliance.

Prozac's lack of side effects and its ability to ameliorate disorders in which tricyclics often fail have led to changes in the way psychiatrists see patients and the way patients see themselves.

Fluoxetine's benign side effects profile is a major factor in promoting compliance; more important in light of data suggesting the need for long-term therapy. Breakthrough symptoms or relapse are less likely to occur with missed doses because of the drug's extended half-life (24 to 72 hours). Early nonresponders usually improve on increasing the dose to 40mg (two capsules) after six weeks. However, the great majority of patients show some improvements in depressive symptomatology within the first week. I noticed that patients were frequently unaware of the early, subtle improvements in their depressive syndrome.

Major depression is an insidious disease that exacts high personal and economic costs. It affects at least 15 million Americans each year and is more common than hypertension in primary care practice. Untreated or inadequately treated, it is a disease associated with high mortality, morbidity and economic costs. The total cost of depression, based on 1980 economic data, is $16.3 billion, of which only a small portion, approximately $2.1 billion, goes to diagnosis and treatment. The remainder—$14.2 billion—falls into the category of indirect costs, such as those to health care system, employers and society. Patients with affective disorders are high utilizers of health care, making approximately three times more visits to health care providers than those who do not suffer from depression.

Many patients with untreated depression received aggressive medical treatment and testing for vague somatic complaints. Furthermore, patients with major depression have five times the risk of disability as compared with nondepressed persons. Successful antidepressant therapy has been found to result in 80% decrease in acute hospital costs.

It can be argued that it is more cost-effective to treat someone suffering from major depression when loss of productivity, loss of employment and the social costs for the depressed person are taken into consideration. There are indications that a number of people suffering from major depression remain undiagnosed and untreated. This is particularly true for masked depression (as I have discussed in Chapter VI entitled MASKED DEPRESSION). These patients present with aches and pains and general malaise, but do not acknowledge being depressed.

Fortunately, depression can be effectively treated and experience has shown that pharmacotherapy was the most effective treatment for moderate to severe depression. As discussed earlier in this introduction, cognitive behavior therapy expedited the recovery from illness which remains a major challenge in general practice.

The World Health Organization at one time, identified depression as a growing and serious problem throughout the world. WHO has since launched a series of studies designed to develop the means to identify depression in different cultures and to better understand its nature. Probably the incidence of depression may not really be increasing. However, the discovery in the early 60's of drugs for the treatment of affective disorders may also have increased our motivation to find and label certain types of disorders as depression. The epidemiology of depression presents, however, a different story. Even if we have not yet been able to establish beyond doubt that depression is on the increase, there are strong reasons why we can expect to see patients with depressive disorders in increasing numbers in the future. First the World Health Organization and the National Institute of Mental Health have been highly insensitive for certain reasons: with the increased life expectancy observed in most countries of the world, the proportion of individuals who are at risk for developing an age-related depressive disorder increases: an increase in morbidity from chronic cardiovascular disease, cerebrovascular and other neurologic disease has been shown to be associated with depressive reactions in as many as 20% of all cases. The WHO sees more and more people in some countries being uprooted with the resultant family disintegration; and in the U.S. rising divorce rates are leading to increasing social isolation among young and middle-aged adults. The stresses of urbanization for primarily poorer populations are expected to increase psychiatric disorders of all types.

Depression is more common in people who have had to make major emotional adjustments in their lives during the past 6-12 months, for example, due to the death of a family member, the birth of a baby, the loss of a job or frequent changes of residence. All these events may result in persistent stress. See later under "Is Stress Worth Worrying About?". Over time, the effects of such stress make you vulnerable to depression. In order to resolve fully the depression and to prevent recurrences it is important to resolve stress. The first priority in tackling stress is to ensure that you are getting sufficient exercise, a nourishing diet and enough sleep.

Much of this book carries practical, in-depth details emphasizing the art of treatment as well as the science. It is important that relatives support the patient in the initial treatment phase of depression. Patients and their relatives increasingly need to be well-informed and in this text I have tried to explain in a simple manner the steps which should be taken in dealing with a disorder which requires compliance from the patient and support from the family.

Depression can affect people of all ages, but severe depression usually begins around the age of 30-40 years. In the beginning, when the onset of depressive illness is fairly sudden, symptoms can develop in one to two weeks, although it is more usual for the rate to be two or three times slower. The most common symptoms are depressed mood, anxiety and loss of interest; sleep difficulties, loss of appetite, lack of energy, fatigue and suicidal thought soon follow. After three to five months, patients tend to seek medical help because they can no longer cope. By this time the illness is often severe, and profoundly depressed mood, guilty thoughts and suicidal ideas are clearly present. In the most severe depressive illness, hallucinations and delusions develop but this is rare. If depressive illness has become established, it tends to last for months, perhaps even years, without treatment. The most important problem is that many patients with depression remain undiagnosed. Every year a doctor will treat many patients for depression but may fail to recognize or to be consulted by quite a number of patients who have concealed depression. (This will be discussed further under the topic Masked Depression).

CONTENTS

Chapter 1

DEPRESSION:
A NATIONAL HEALTH PROBLEM

UNDERSTANDING MOOD DISORDERS

Depression is one of the most prevalent emotional disorders. Because depression is so common and can be so debilitating, much effort has been devoted to determining the cause. Depressive illness is a persistent exaggeration of the everyday feelings that accompany sadness. It is a disturbance of mood, of variable severity and duration, that is frequently recurrent, and accompanied by a variety of physical and mental symptoms, involving thinking, life and judgement. Depression is usually recognized by the affected individual or close family and friends when the symptoms become severe or last for too long.

Studies have found that as many as 30% of primary care patients are clinically depressed. Initial surveys found that nearly one half of all office visits for a mental illness are to non-psychiatrists, specially the primary care physicians and internists. Some of these patients have major depression, a few severe cases are referred to as psychotic depression, and others show less-than-frank major depression with either dysthymia or so-called "subsyndromal" depressive symptoms. The frequency of presentation of patients with clinical depression at the primary care physicians office is in sharp contrast to the frequency of the diagnosis of the patient made in this same patient. One study found that less than 50% of depressed patients were actually diagnosed as such. Worse, only a small fraction (only 5%) of the half that were diagnosed actually received adequate treatment. This means that the large numbers of patients with clinical depression are left in a state of continued morbid dysfunction, thus increasing the potential for suicide. Also, these patients continued to be frequent users of medical care and therefore are a major factor in hampering the cost-effectiveness of medical care. Consequently, it behoves the primary care practitioner and other non-psychiatrists to be acutely aware of and knowledgeable about the diagnosis of this *highly treatable disease.*

We will now look briefly at several approaches to understanding affective disorders.

Psychoanalytic Perspective: Psychoanalytic theories interpret the depression as the *reaction to loss*. Whatever the nature of loss (loss of a loved one, loss of status, loss of moral support provided by a group of friends), the depressed person reacts to it intensely because the current situation brings back all the feelings of an earlier loss that occurred in childhood—that being the loss of parental affection. For some reason, the individual's needs for affection were not satisfied in childhood. A loss in later life causes the individual to regress to his or her hopeless, dependent state when the original loss occurred. Part of the depressed person's behavior, therefore, represents a cry for love—a display of hopelessness and an appeal for affection and security. The reaction to loss is complicated by angry feelings towards the deserting person. An underlying assumption of psychoanalytic theories that people who are prone to depression have learned to repress their hostile feelings because they are afraid of alienating those on whom they depend for support. When things go wrong, they turn to anger and blame themselves. Psychoanalytical theories suggest that the depressed person's low self-esteem and feelings of worthlessness stem from a childhood need for parental approval. The self-esteem of a person prone to depression depends primarily on external sources; the approval of others. When these supports fail, then the individual may be left in the state of depression.

Behavioral Perspective: Learning theorists assume that lack of reinforcement plays a major role in depression. The inactivity of the depressed person and the feelings of sadness are due to a low rate of positive reinforcement and/or a high rate of unpleasant experiences. Many of the events that precipitate depression (such as the death of a loved one, loss of job or impaired health) reduce accustomed reinforcement. As people become depressed and inactive, their main source of reinforcement is the sympathy and attention they receive from relatives and friends. This attention may initially reinforce the varied behaviors that are maladaptive (weeping, complaining, criticizing themselves, talking about suicide). But because it is tiresome to be around someone who refuses to cheer up, the depressed person's behavior eventually alienates even those close associates, producing a further reduction in reinforcement and increasing the individual's social assimilation and unhappiness.

Cognitive Perspective: Cognitive theories of depression focuses not on what people do but on how they view themselves and the world. One of the more influential cognitive theories, developed by Aaron Beck, is derived from extensive therapeutic experience with depressed patients. Beck's theory suggests that individuals prone to depression have developed a general attitude of appraising events from a negative and self-critical viewpoint. They expect to fail rather than to succeed, and they tend to magnify failures and minimize successes in evaluating their performance.

Another cognitive approach to depression, developed by Martin Seligman, derives from experiments on *learned helplessness*. According to this theory, people become depressed when they *believe* that their actions make no difference in bringing about either pleasure or pain. Depression is caused by the expectation of future helplessness. A depressed person expects bad events to occur and believes that there is nothing he or she can do to prevent them from happening.

The theories of Beck and Seligman have stimulated a great deal of research on the cognitive processes of depressed individuals, and the results have demonstrated that self-critical attitudes and attributions of helplessness are important components of depression. This issue will be discussed fully in Chapter X called COGNITIVE BEHAVIOR THERAPY.

Biological Perspective: A tendency to develop mood disorders, particularly bipolar disorders (also known as manic-depression), appears to be inherited. These conditions in the individual alternates between depression and normal mood and between extreme elation and normal mood. In some cases, the cycle between depressive episodes and manic episodes is swift with only a brief return to normality in between. The specific role that genetic factors play in mood disorders is far from clear. However, it seems likely that a biochemical abnormality is involved. Mounting evidence indicates that our moods are regulated by *neurotransmitters*, that transmit nerve impulses from one neuron to another. A number of chemicals serve as neurotransmitters in different parts of the brain and normal behavior requires a careful balance among them. This will be discussed fully in Chapter V.

The most important problem is that many patients with depression remain undiagnosed, and one of the aims of this book is to help to increase the rate of accurate diagnosis of depression by general practitioners. Every year a general practitioner will treat about 30 patients for depression but may fail to recognize or be consulted by ten times as many patients who have concealed depression. Patients and their relatives increasingly need to be well-informed and this text with its simple approach could prove to be helpful in a disorder which requires compliance from the patient and support from the family. About half the patients on antidepressants do not take the medication as prescribed and most of them will have stopped taking altogether within a few weeks, sometimes because of side-effects, but often because they do not understand the mode of action of the drug or length of treatment required. The main areas in which family doctors' management of depression can be improved are the prescription of adequate doses of antidepressant, patient treatment compliance, patient supervision and recognition of the patient with organic diseases. The older tricyclic antidepressants have side-effects which also increase the frequency of non-compliance.

That's why the new generation antidepressant such as Prozac with no side-effects are more popular among the patients.

TYPES OF DEPRESSION

Depression has been classified as endogenous or exogenous (reactive) in origin, and as psychotic or neurotic. Anxiety is more difficult to categorize, since the term is often used to describe any unpleasant mood. Anxiety is generally characterized by feelings of foreboding and feeling of danger or harm, with accompanying similar symptoms, and all precipitating environmental influence. The ability to diagnose and classify the depressive illnesses more accurately has been accompanied by a greater specificity of available therapies (See Chapter V). In the past, depression has been subdivided into "reactive" depression, i.e. occurs in response to adversity, and "endogenous" depression, which was thought to be unrelated to the environment or circumstances. These terms are gradually being replaced by neurotic (instead of reactive), and psychotic (instead of endogenous). This is because depressed patients are classified according to the symptoms that they display (i.e. neurotic symptoms or psychotic symptoms), whereas the older terms refer to the causation. Endogenous depression is defined in terms of sadness, social withdrawal, loss of libido, anorexia/weight loss, retardation/agitation, early morning awakening, guilt, loss of pleasure, and mood unresponsive to the environment. This mood is qualitatively distinct from normal sadness.

Depression is sometimes a prominent part of an anxiety syndrome, but there are many, even in severely anxious patients, who do not show any depression. However, in the long run, anxious patients often become moody, and episodes of severe depression are not rare. Panic disorders and agoraphobia are particularly often complicated by depression and also by alcohol or drug dependence. Anxiety disorders tend to restrict the patient's social sphere and make many activities difficult and laborious. Affective disorders and anxiety disorders seem to share some biological mechanisms. In depression there is always an element of anxiety, and anxiety states often give rise to secondary depression, if a depressive element is not there from the beginning. Most of these elements can be present in about the same proportion, preventing a clear differential diagnosis. During periods of depression, phobic and/or obsessive phenomena often emerge, to disappear again after the cure of depression. In such cases, the diagnosis is not a phobia or obsessive/compulsive disorder. In schizophrenia, anxiety is often present, and obsessive/compulsive phenomena are quite common. Such partial phenomena should not be mistaken for genuine anxiety or for obsessive/compulsive disorder. Anxiety disorders, especially the more chronic ones like obsessive/compulsive disorder, may involve more or less of a depressive element, often of a secondary nature. In diagnostic rating as well as in treatment of such disorders, it is wise also to consider the degree of depression.

Why is the incidence of depression increasing?

Actually, the incidence of depression may *not* really be increasing. It is possible that the professions have simply, for various reasons, increased their sensitivity, or begun to utilize methods not available in the past for its detection which make it appear more prevalent. The discovery in the early 60's of drugs for the treatment of affective disorders may also have increased our motivation to find and label certain types of disorders as depression. Such disorders were not called depression before the availability of effective treatments. It is not the first time that this has happened in medicine. Most investigators would agree, e.g. that there is no evidence that the extent of mania has significantly increased in the world. Yet proportionately more of mania is diagnosed now than 20 years ago. We attribute that increase in diagnosed cases to the discovery of lithium, and effective, specific treatment for that clinicians (the availability of lithium apparently raised the awareness of conditions to manic-like symptoms in patients suffering from a range of disorders). The epidemiology of depression presents, however, a different story. Even if we have not yet been able to establish beyond doubt that it is on the increase, there are strong reasons why we can expect to see patients with depressive disorders in increasing numbers in the future.

Both the World Health Organization and the National Institute of Mental Health have been highly sensitive to certain of these reasons:

1. With the increased life expectancy observed in most countries of the world, the proportion of individuals who are at risk for developing an age-related depressive disorder increases;
2. An increase in mobility from chronic cardiovascular diseases, cerebro-vascular and other neurological diseases has been shown to be associated with depressive reactions in as many as 20% of all cases;
3. The rapidly changing psychosocial environment of man, which often gives rise to situations of acute or prolonged environmental stress, may lead to an increase in depressive reactions. The WHO, for example, sees more and more people in some countries being uprooted with family disintegration.

Some additional factors that have been found to increase vulnerability to depression include having fewer social skills, being poor, being very dependent on others, having children under the age of seven, and not having a close and intimate confidante. The last of these appears to be the most important, at least for women, since it has been the most consistently identified over various studies. Having an intimate, confiding relation with a husband or a friend decreases the risk of a woman becoming depressed when confronted with a stressful life situation. This is consistent with the research which indicates that social supports reduce the severity of stressful events. Thus, depression has many causes, which may range from being determined almost entirely by an inherited biochemical abnormality to being exclusively the result of psychological or environmental factors. Most cases fall in between the two extremes and involve a mixture of genetic, early developmental, and environmental factors.

Depressive illness is a persistent exaggeration of the everyday feelings that accompany sadness. Depression is usually recognized by the affected individual or close family and friends when the symptoms become severe or last far too long. In practice, established depressive illness is recognized by listing several of the following symptoms: sleep disturbance; persistent, low, miserable mood; a lack of enjoyment or pleasure in the usual activities. Also, there is reduced energy and weariness; loss of appetite or weight; impaired efficiency; guilt; inability to concentrate and make decisions; distinctive posture and gesture.

In severe depression, the above characteristics are present with greater intensity and may be accompanied by suicidal ideation, plans or acts; tendency to drink; delusions and/or hallucinations. In a primary care setting, the goal should be to recognize and treat incipient depression very quickly. The longer a patient's depression persists, especially when it is experienced daily, the more likely it is that depressive illness is present. Most episodes of depression lasting for more than two weeks become depressive illnesses. Depression can affect people of all ages, but severe depression usually begins at around the age of 30-40 years.

The most disastrous consequence of depression is suicide. Of the reported 25,000 people who end their lives by suicide in the U.S. every year, the majority are suffering from depression. However, suicide deaths are under-reported for a variety of reasons. Because of the stigma attached to suicide, physicians and coroners may be persuaded by the family to list the death as accidental when the circumstances are questionable. Women attempt to commit suicide about three times more often than men, but men succeed in killing themselves more often than women. The greater number of suicide attempts by women is probably related to the greater incidence of depression among women. The fact that men are more successful in their attempts is related to the choice of method. Among the reasons most frequently cited by those who have attempted suicide are depression, loneliness, ill-health, marital problems, and financial or job difficulties. The greatest number of suicides occur among people in their fifties, and the rate continues to be high through age 60 and over. Recently, however, suicide has increased among adolescents and young adults. In fact, the incidence of suicide among 15-24 year olds in the U.S. has almost tripled over the last two decades. Suicidal college students, on average, have higher records of academic achievement than their non-suicidal classmates, whereas most adolescents who commit suicide have exceptionally poor high school records. The adolescents tend to be dropouts or to have behavioral problems in school. The outstanding characteristic of adolescents who attempt suicide due to social isolation: they describe themselves as loners, most have parents who were divorced or separated, a large number also have alcoholic parents, and in most cases, were not living at home at the time of their suicide attempt.

Another factor contributing to suicide, in addition to depression, is drug abuse. However, most people who commit suicide acts are experiencing such turmoil and stress that their thinking is far from clear. They are not sure whether they want to live or die; they want to do both at the same time, e.g. one more than the other. Since the best predictor of a future suicide is a prior attempt, all parasuicides (attempted suicide) should be taken seriously. Few people commit suicide without signalling their intention to someone. Thus, a person who talks about suicide may actually attempt it. Many communities have established suicide-prevention centres where troubled individuals can seek help, either through telephone contact or in person.

Suicide is a major preventable cause of death; at least 50% of those who commit suicide signal their intention to their doctor. The majority has seen their family doctor (75% in the month before suicide and 50% in the week before; 25% have seen a psychiatrist, 50% in the week before their death); 80% have been prescribed psychotropic drugs (Wilkinson; '89). Virtually all were mentally ill; 70% were suffering from depression and 15% from alcoholism. Physicians must also be alert to signs of depression in motor vehicle accident-prone adolescents, since accidents may represent "MASKED" suicide attempts in adolescent to verbalize his feelings and careful interviewing may identify feelings of hopelessness and assess suicide risk. The professional should inquire about suicide risk in a direct manner (Hancock and Walker; '90).

Assessment of the suicide risk is one of the most difficult of the doctor's tasks, for a patient who is set on taking his life is sometimes likely to conceal his intention so as not to have it thwarted. This dilemma has prompted the development of a special method of assessing suicidal tendencies. Given the reduced level of risk by the young, in the case of a patient living in a family environment where there is always someone to care for him, while the same risk would appear excessive in, say, a patient living alone in some solitary room without human contacts. The success of **prophylactic** treatment further demands that the subject of suicide should not be **taboo**, but the doctor and patient should be able to discuss the matter **frankly** . Agitation and acute suicidal tendency should initially be treated with a neuroleptic with a potent sedative effect, even when the patient is depressed. Once sedation has been achieved, and even perhaps in combination with the neuroleptic, antidepressant therapy can be instituted. In depression with milder suicidal tendencies it is judicious to use antidepressants with calming properties, since those with a disinhibiting, activating effect may intensify or provoke anxiety, agitation and suicidal tendencies. A further important point is that it is inadvisable to treat suicidal patients with predominantly mood-elevating antidepressants alone, since they invariably have more than a mild sedative effect and require days or even weeks to achieve their actual antidepressant action. The suicidal impulse, on the other hand, must be countered **at once**. Such cases call for administration of antidepressants with a calming effect, or a combination of predominantly mood-elevating antidepressants with neuroleptic.

When the patient improves, it may be necessary to see the patient weekly to begin with, then, when progress is satisfactory, every two weeks, and, finally, mostly for three to six months. However, it is usually advisable to inform the patient and any relatives that they should contact the doctor at any time if they are worried. It is also advisable to continue to see the patient monthly for two to three months once they have recovered to check for signs of *relapse*. Specialist help may be required for patients in whom the diagnosis is in doubt, there is a high risk of suicide being attempted or progress is slow despite appropriate treatment. The majority of disturbed patients, in particular, those who have psychological or motor retardation, agitation or psychotic symptoms, such as hallucinations and delusion, will need to be referred to a psychiatrist. In disturbed patients, the illness is obvious to all concerned, including relatives, who are often pleased to have specialist advice and treatment. Patients with depression who live alone, or take excess alcohol, are also particularly vulnerable and usually require extra social support as part of their treatment.

Doctors have particular problems in dealing with old people with depression. Affective disorders are common in the elderly, and are distressing, not only for the sufferers themselves, but also for their families and supporters. Diagnosis is difficult, since the characteristic symptoms of depression may be less prominent in old people, or may be attributed to the normal aging or co-existent physical disease. Since old age is often a time of loss and unhappiness, it is sometimes difficult to decide whether sadness is a realistic response to unfortunate circumstances or a pathological condition requiring drug therapy. Treatment is made more difficult by the fact that old people are more likely to be intolerant of antidepressant compounds, which are metabolized more slowly in the elderly. Cardiovascular disorders are specially common in patients with depression, and may cause particular sensitivity to antidepressants. While safety and efficacy of the tricyclic antidepressant (TCAs) in low doses are established in the fit elderly, considerable doubts remain over whether TCAs are effective and safe in the medically ill. While there is smaller volume of research on fit young adults, there is more adequate research on the use of such drugs as the new Prozac for the elderly depressed to reach firm conclusion about both safety and efficacy. This is more effective treatment than TCAs and has significant advantage as it produces fewer side effects, particularly fewer anticholinergic effects such as dry mouth, constipation, blurred vision, etc., which often cause treatment termination in the elderly because of promoting confusional states as well.

Although prevalence is not definitely established, one report suggests that about 15% of elderly individuals living in the community have substantial dysphoria and that 4% have major depressive disorders. Unfortunately, physicians and patients alike frequently consider depression an inevitable concomitant of aging, and they believe that depression is inherent to aging as often it resulted in patients in failing to seek treatment, and in physicians providing minimum diagnostic and therapeutic attention. These attitudes result in a prognosis. Many people feel that no matter what is done, a third get better, a third stay the same, and a third get worse. However, pessimism surrounding prognosis in the elderly is unwarranted. Depression is the most easily treated functional disorder of old age, and prompt and appropriate intervention can restore the mental health of a geriatric individual, particularly now with the new generation antidepressants.

Pitfalls include considering sadness, dysphoria inherent to the aging process, mistaken depression for organic brain syndrome or physical disease, or assuming a functional disorder when illness or drug interaction is the culprit.

Also, the elderly are usually taking several medications and some of them have been implicated in depression, (such as antipsychotics, L-Dopa, and antihypertensive medications such as propranolol).

Unfortunately, depression all too often seems ubiquitous affecting at least 10% of Western industrialized population. Samples of most communities will attain diagnoses of severe illness in 5%, value rising to 10-20% through adulthood and up to fully 33% of persons in Nursing Homes. The female:male sex ratio in unipolar depressed patients is about 2:1. Clinical (unipolar) depression is so widespread that it has been called "the common cold" of psychiatry (Seligman; '75). At any given point in time, 15-20% of adults suffer significant levels of depressive symptomatology. At least 12% experience depression severe enough to require treatment at some time in their lives, and depression has been estimated to account for 75% of psychiatric hospitalization.

Several years ago as part of a national report, Katz at the National Institute of Mental Health (NIMH) reviewed the status of research on the depressive disorder. Then he noted in 1973 that for the mental health professionals these disorders had begun to rival schizophrenia in the sheer magnitude of the problem and in their consequent demand on services. Further, in reviewing the results of a survey on the pattern of psychotropic drug use in the USA, it turned out that upwards of 30% of the general population was reporting significant psychiatric distress, and that fully half of this group acknowledge symptomatology of primarily depressive nature. The 15% population figure was not an isolated statistic but apparently it was replicated in at least two other similar studies.

There is apparently another group of the population, which needs further study and possibly clinical assessment in meeting their life problems. All these figures have been under continuing surveillance by the World Health Organization, which, has since launched a series of studies designed to develop the means to identify depression in different cultures and to better understand its nature.

Major depressive disorder is an insidious disease that exacts high personal and economic costs. It affects at least 15 million Americans each year, and is more common than hypertension in primary care practise. Untreated or inadequately treated, it is a disease associated with high mortality, morbidity, and economic costs.

For reasons as yet unclear, the rate of depression among women in western industrialized nations is approximately twice the rate among men. It seems likely that no single factor can explain the occurrence of depression, but rather that it results from an interaction between many different factors. Its onset and course have been shown to relate to a variety of biological, historical, environmental and psychosocial variables. These include (as would be explained in Chapter IV) disturbances in neurotransmitter functioning, a family history of depression or alcoholism, early parental loss or neglect, recent negative life events, lack of a close, confiding relationship, lack of adequate social support, and a long-term lack of self esteem.

When people become clinically depressed, they feel sad, and are often tearful. They are troubled by guilt, believing that they are letting people down. They may become more irritable than usual, more anxious and tense. When the depression is at its worst, they may lose the ability to react emotionally, and find that good and bad feelings alike are lost in numbness. It becomes difficult to enjoy or be interested in normal activities. Energy is low and everything seems an effort. So they tend to withdraw from the things they would normally do, and spend long hours hunched in a chair or lying in bed.

Although effective pharmacologic therapy has been available for nearly 40 years, most patients have been treated inadequately. The side effects associated with available antidepressants usually led to sub-therapeutic dosing, premature discontinuation of therapy, or lack of patient compliance. The introduction in 1988 of Prozac (Fluoxetine), the first selective serotonin uptake inhibitor (SSUI) or selective serotonin re-uptake inhibitor (SSRI) available in the United States, represented a major advance in the pharmacological management of depression.

In the past, 15% of patients with major depressive disorders commit suicide.

Impact on quality of life is substantial. A study of more than 11,000 outpatients revealed that the well-being and physical function of a patient with major depression or depressive symptoms was worse than that of patient with chronic medical conditions including hypertension, arthritis, diabetes, and back pain; only patients with current heart conditions scored lower than patients with depressive symptoms. The combination of depression and another medical condition exerted an additive effect, further worsening physical functioning.

Although depressive illness is very common, its extent varies in different places and in different groups. Surveys show that 20-30% of the population may suffer symptoms of depression in the course of one year. Most cases are mild but about one person in 20 will have moderate or severe episodes. Severe depression affects about 4% of the population, but only one fifth of this group would seek medical treatment. It is believed that about one in 50 depressives need hospital treatment. The incidence of depression is lower in married people than in single people; among women, the incidence and prevalence of depression varies with ages—the highest rate occur in the 34-45 years age-group. Women are about twice as likely as men to suffer from mild depression, but for severe depression and recurrent depression equal proportions of men and women suffer. The rates of depression increase with age in men.

Depression is a major challenge to general practice. It has an uncomfortable mortality and every year in an average group practice at least one successful suicide occurs which is potentially preventable. Depression has been estimated to account for 75% of psychiatric hospitalization.

Many, many millions of people throughout the world suffer from mild degrees of tension and depression. Only a few of them will ever see a psychiatrist. Far too often we hear the expression, "you must learn to live with it". This is not good enough. That is why it is very important that the patient, particularly if he is suffering from moderate to severe depression, must be treated properly with either cognitive behavioral therapy or with this very effective medication, Prozac. Cognitive behavioral assessment is based on simple principles and has clearly defined ends. The first, and perhaps central principle of cognitive behavioral assessment is that the ways in which an individual behaves are determined by immediate situations and the individual's interpretation of them. This therefore becomes the major focus of the assessment, with an emphasis on specific problems rather than global entities.

The goal of the therapy is to find solutions to the patients' problems, using cognitive-behavioral strategies, not merely to help the patient think more "rationally". The immediate target is symptom-relief. At this stage an antidepressant such as Prozac is appropriate and should always be considered early in the treatment.

Appropriate treatment for depression may substantially lower health-care costs as well as mortality and morbidity. Successful antidepressant therapy has been found to result in an almost 80% decrease in acute hospital costs. Effective treatment also counteracts the loss of workplace productivity commonly associated with depression. Data based on 1980 costs indicate that approximately five million work days and 10 billion dollars are lost annually in America due to depression.

Peter Stokes ('93) believes that the total annual cost of depression is 16.3 billion dollars of which only a small portion, approximately 2.1 billion dollars goes to diagnosis and treatment. The remainder—that is 14.2 billion dollars—falls in to the category of indirect costs, such as those to the Health Care System, employers, and society. Patients with affective disorders are high utilizers of health care, making approximately three times more visits to health-care providers than those who do not suffer from depression. Furthermore, patients with major depression have five times the risk of disability as compared with non-depressed persons.

Fortunately, depression can be effectively treated. It has been shown that pharmacotherapy was the most effective treatment for moderate to severe depression. Pharmacotherapy and psychotherapy were equally effective in the management of mild depression but recovery was more rapid with pharmacotherapy.

Chapter 2

MENTAL ILLNESSES ARE NOT CAUSED BY BAD PARENTING OR BAD "SPOUSING"

Traditional psychoanalysis emphasized fear of the domineering father in fostering inferiority. Psychoanalysts have deemed low self-esteem to result from failures in parental empathy. Constantly critical parents do often destroy the confidence of their children. There has been a great deal of research which points to the role of parenting in the formation of self-esteem. Self-esteem in young children correlates with measures of parental warmth, acceptance and respect. Low self-esteem is so closely related to depressed mood, social inhibition and reactivity. People with low self-esteem often say or believe bad things about themselves, and many people with low self-esteem were taught in childhood that they are inferior to others.

Guilt: it strikes at everyone—except, maybe, psychopaths. It can be a powerful force—whether constructive or destructive. People feel guilty about almost anything: their deception, their aggression, their lack of sympathy for others, and more importantly, about the way they brought up their children. The degree to which guilt is experienced will often depend upon cultural and religious aspects. Members of family and community-oriented cultures may not regard themselves as individually responsible for their actions. But in Western societies, where **individuality** is openly encouraged, guilt is more likely to be present. Americans, Australians and English are particularly susceptible to guilt because individualism is emphasized.

Guilt is the punishing voice of an authority figure or the parent within. We feel guilty when we think we haven't measured up to our own or someone else's unreal expectations. It takes roots in our childhood and can sometimes hound us to old age.

Nowadays, parents are feeling guilty because both father and mother are working. In an era looking for reassurance that two-career households are not harmful to children, parents are reading Dr. Benjamin Spock's book, but then also trying to reconcile it with the ideas of Penelope Leach, Britain's leading authority on child rearing. At the heart of Leach philosophy is the labor-intensive—and guilt-inducing—conviction that adults can never be there enough for their kids. Her books—especially her 1977 standard *Baby and Child*, which sold more than three million copies worldwide—have done well. (Dr. Spock's *Baby and Child Care*, far ahead at 40 million, has the advantage of more than 45 years in print). Not bad for a woman who appears to believe that there's hardly a parent who makes the grade.

Leach believes that mothers should be at home—not in the workplace—during early childhood: "The more you are around, the better", counsels Leach. She continues to say: "Our assumption is always that we should handle babies in the way that costs us least time. The last thing we want to do is keep on being interrupted in our adult affairs to chat to them or cuddle them or whatever". In her latest book, *Children First*, she moves on to a wider-ranging critique of the workplace, government policies and legal systems for failing to give first priority to the presumed best interests of children. As for day care, there is of course a great dilemma. In the U.S., for example, nearly 70% of women with children work; her critics complain that she disregards the fact that most do so out of economic necessity. Most families, nowadays, need women's income to survive; there just isn't enough income otherwise. They also criticize her for leaving the impression that children raised in day care will suffer.

Leach's book expands upon her controversial notion that day care is a grave mistake for kids under three. "The more you are around, the better; and the younger the child, the more it matters". She encourages mothers to stay at home at least until they have seen their brood through childhood. She is of the opinion that if you give even five or ten years to this child-centered way of life, there is still an awful lot of time for you to be you. She takes positions on discipline that can make the famously permissive Dr. Spock seem a despot by comparison. There's nothing for either of you in not leaving on the light, she tells readers, as a way to deal with children who won't sleep without one. "If you look to the child, the answer is perfectly clear and simple". Convinced that spanking interferes with a child's developing self-discipline, Leach is a leading figure in a British campaign to turn public opinion against it. "It has aroused enormous controversy because physical punishment is regarded as a parental right", she admits.

Infants differ from one another in the degree to which they form attachments to their primary caregivers in the first year of life. The failure to form secure attachments in the early years has been related to an inability to develop close personal relationships in adulthood. After the first year of a child's life, childrearing becomes more complex as parents take on the trickier task of discipline, control, and character building. Parents differ markedly from one another in how they approach these tasks. Some are warm, nurturing, and relaxed; others are cold, aloof, and tense. Some are highly controlling, others tend to let the children do their own thing. Some are **child-centered**, highly involved in their children's lives; others are parent-centered, more occupied with their own interests and activities.

A basic task for psychology is to categorize and summarize these many differences and to determine if and how they help shape the child's personality. Parents who combine control with acceptance and child-centered involvement are called **authoritative**. They exercise a high level of control and require their children to behave at intellectual and social levels consistent with their age and abilities. But authoritative parents combine their control and demands with warmth, nurturance and two-way communication. They solicit their children's opinions and feelings when family decisions are made, and they offer explanations and reasons for punitive or restrictive measures whenever they feel these must be imposed. Children of such parents tend to be independent, self-assertive, friendly with peers, and co-operative with parents. They are also likely to be successful both intellectually and socially. They seem to enjoy life; and they have strong motivation to achieve.

Controlling and demanding parents who simply assert their power without warmth, nurturance, or two-way communication are labelled **authoritarian**. They attempt to control and evaluate the behavior and attitude of their children in accordance with absolute set of standards. They also value obedience, respect for authority, work, tradition and preservation of order. Children of such parents tend to be moderately competent and responsible, but they also tend to be socially withdrawn and to lack spontaneity. The girls seem to be particularly dependent on their parents and lacking in achievement and motivation; the boys tend to be more aggressive than other boys. Some studies also find a link between authoritarian parenting and low self-esteem in boys.

A recent study conducted in Finland assessed the children of **parent-centered** parents. Compared with children of child-centered parents, children of parent-centered parents at age 14 were impulsive; they lacked concentration, were moody, spent money quickly rather than saving it, and had difficulty controlling aggressive outbursts. They were uninterested in school, likely to be truant, and spent time dating at earlier ages.

However, the results on childbearing practices and children's personalities are reasonably consistent but they are fairly weak. In fact, they are much weaker than many researchers had expected. Some psychologists are even coming to believe that, in general, differences between families have little to do with differences in children's personalities. This startling conclusion, hence the title of this chapter: "Mental illnesses are not caused by bad parenting".

In shaping personality, genetic and environmental influences do not act independently of one another but are intertwined from the moment of birth. Parents give their biological offspring both their genes and a home environment, and both are functions of the parents' own genes. As a result, there is a built-in correlation between the child's own inherited characteristics (genotype) and his or her environment. For example, because general intelligence is partially heritable, parents with high intelligence are likely to have children with high intelligence. But parents with high intelligence are also likely to provide an intellectually stimulating environment for their children—both through their own interactions with them and through books, piano lessons, trips to museums, etc. Because the child's genes and environment are positively correlated in this way, he or she will get a double-dose of intellectual advantage.

THE ASSOCIATIONS BETWEEN LIFE PROBLEMS AND EMOTIONAL DISORDERS

Are certain types of mental illness more likely to be caused by specific psychosocial stresses than others? Do certain mild adaptive behaviors occur circumventing to mental illness as a form of psychosocial handicap? If either of these reactions occurs, do they happen separately or together? For the last two decades, there has been a great deal of psychosocial research on psycho pathology. This has tended to be concerned with the structural basis of psychiatric illnesses, such as sex, social class and race. These investigations have moved towards the examination of a "vulnerability model" for psychiatric disorders. This model presupposes that there are certain factors in individuals or the immediate environment that lead them to decompensate in the case of different levels of stresses. It is concluded that patients who develop chronic psychiatric illnesses are probably more psychologically or are biologically vulnerable than those patients who develop short-lived disorders and who do not achieve a major psychiatric illness.

MOOD DISORDERS

Mood refers to the internal emotional state of one individual; *affect*, to the external expression of emotional content. There are psychological conditions of mood and affect, the most serious of which are the mood disorders, depression and mania. Depression and mania are called affective disorders in DSM-III; in DSM-III-R, they are grouped together as mood disorders. Mood may be normal, elevated, or depressed. A normal individual expresses a wide range of moods and has an equally large repertoire of affective expressions; he feels in control of his moods and affects. Mood disorders are a group of clinical conditions characterized by a disturbance of mood, loss of that sense of control, and a subjective experience of great distress. Patients with an elevated mood demonstrate extensive flight of ideas, decreased sleep, heightened self-esteem and grandiose ideas. On the other hand, patients with depressed mood show loss of energy and interest, guilt feelings, difficulty in concentrating, loss of appetite, and thoughts of death or suicide.

Other signs and symptoms include decreasing activity level, cognitive abilities, speech and vegetative functions (e.g. sleep, appetite, sexual activity, and other biological reasons). These disorders virtually always result in impaired interpersonal, social, and occupational function.

Patients who are afflicted only with major depressive episodes are said to have major depressive disorders, or **unipolar depression**. A patient who has both manic and depressive episodes or a patient with manic episodes alone are said to have **bipolar disorder**. The terms unipolar mania and pure mania are sometimes used for bipolar patients who do not have depressive episodes. The field of psychiatry has considered unipolar depression and bipolar disorder to be two separate disorders, particularly in the last 20 years. However, reconsideration has been given more recently to the possibility that bipolar disorder is actually a more severe expression of a unipolar depression. Another trend in psychiatry has been to consider depression and mania as two ends of a continuum of emotional experience. This concept is not supported by the common clinical with observation that many patients have mixed states with both depressed and manic features.

Psychiatry, a branch of medicine, is responsible for the study, diagnosis, treatment, and prevention of human behavior disorders. Abnormal behavior may be determined or modified by genetic, physicochemical, psychological and social factors as mentioned above. The psychiatrist must muster the knowledge and skills not only of objective observation, but also subjective, participant, and self observation. His background in natural science has fostered objective observation, but as he learns other types, he finds this, added differentiation of his role function is necessary for understanding the relationship to his patient and for his growth in his capacity for human intimacy. Only then can the general notion of personality and its underlying principles be learned; a genetic and ontogenetic factors in growth, development and decline; a recognition of unconscious and preconscious factors as determinants of behavior and the idea that the personality is integral and indivisible.

We talk about the increased stress of modern living and many nervous breakdowns are attributed to this. Somehow, this implies that the 'good old days' were better than the present time but this simply is not true so far as psychiatric illness is concerned. No doubt many people do become ill as a result of the strains of everyday life, but probably no more than they ever did. However, when a nervous breakdown does occur there is a much greater chance nowadays that the individual would be recognized to be ill and that something positive will be done for him. Until comparatively recently there was virtually no effective treatment for nervous or mental illness. The public at large knew this and also knew the dreadful stigma attached to anyone who had to enter a mental hospital. The result was a natural determination to avoid admission to a mental hospital and thus, if someone was admitted, it was either because he was so deranged or so incapable that he could no longer care for himself in the community, or else because he was a menace to himself or others. The situation has changed radically now and it is obvious that there are very many people who suffer from psychiatric conditions which could never be construed as insanity yet which cause an untold amount of distress to the sufferer. If life is hard and if physical disease and early death are rampant, possibly emotional and psychological disorders appear comparatively unimportant. But in some countries the conditions of life have improved enormously and many people now have both the opportunity to consider the quality of their existence and the material means to enjoy it. If their ability to be happy is affected by excessive anxiety, depression, unreasonable fears or some other psychiatric disability, they are much less likely than before to tolerate this. They will complain and, for the first time, they will expect that something positive should be done about their psychotic complaint.

The psychiatrist is no longer just a custodian of mental illness out of sight of society which finds it distasteful. He has to be in a highly-trained and versatile position with many forms of treatment ready to hand. His speciality becomes one of the more important growth points in modern medical treatment and research.

The whole pattern of psychiatry has changed in recent years. Already, many mental diseases due to physical causes have practically been eradicated in Western countries. For example, mental degeneration due to delayed effects of syphilis used to be common but has become largely preventable since antibiotics were discovered. Epilepsy, which often used to be associated with mental disorders, is much less of a psychiatry problem since the appearance of more sophisticated drug—therapies.

Severe illnesses such as endogenous depression and schizophrenia occur as often today as ever before, but the degree of chronic disability consequent on them has been greatly reduced by modern treatment. Prolonged stays in hospital for these mental conditions are largely a thing of the past and the psychiatric hospitals are rapidly being emptied of their huge population of chronically ill patients. If a mentally ill person has some residual disability he can usually continue to have his treatment in the community, provided that adequate social support is given.

The great majority of patients with psychiatric disorders can increasingly expect to receive good treatment from their general practitioner or at psychiatric outpatient departments. For the minority who require inpatient treatment, the stay in hospital is usually brief and the new policy is to provide treatment in general hospitals and not in a mental hospitals. Psychotic illness is illness, not some dreadful moral lapse. Its stigma is fast disappearing and the more that people realize this and come forward with their problems at an early stage, the more rapidly and completely can we help them. Not so very long ago, books on psychiatric illness would have concentrated on the breakdown rather than on the recovery aspects of mental illness. However, fortunately nowadays, with the discovery of the psychoactive drugs which include the very effective anti-depressant medications, such as Prozac, allows a book like this one to describe confidently the recovery from emotional disorders.

CLASSIFICATION AND DIAGNOSIS OF MENTAL DISEASES

In all medical disciplines, classification of diseases is a dynamic process, ever-changing to incorporate new knowledge. Access to the brain, areas (for measuring and evaluating its function, particularly mental activities), is limited because our understanding of the cause of mental disorders is scant. Since diagnosis implies prognosis and determines choices of therapy, and since standardization of diagnostic categories is essential to research and design, then the need for division of psychiatric nomenclature and classification has been great.

The American Psychiatric Association introduced a new *Diagnostic and Statistical Manual of Mental Disorders* (DSM-I) in 1952. The third edition (DSM-III) was published in 1980 and revised as DSM-III-R in 1987.

Diagnostic Criteria for Depression (adapted from DSM-IV; '94)

At least five of the symptoms listed below should present during the same two week period, most of them occurring nearly every day, representing a change from previous functioning. At least one of the symptoms should be either depressed mood or loss of interest or pleasure. Symptoms which are due to physical condition, mood-incongruent delusions - or hallucinations, or incoherence are not included.

Symptoms:
The major symptoms are shown below.
1. Depressed mood.
2. Markedly diminished interest or pleasure in all activities.
3. Significant weight (loss or weight gain).
4. Insomnia or hyperinsomnia nearly every day.
5. Psychomotor agitation or retardation.
6. Fatigue or loss of energy.
7. Feelings of worthlessness or excessive guilt.
8. Diminished ability to think or concentrate.
9. Recurrence of thoughts of death or suicidal ideation.

During the mental status examination, the classic presentation of a depressed patient is that of a stooped posture with no spontaneous movements and a downcast, averted gaze. Depressed patients commonly have a negative feel of the world and of themselves. About 50-75% of the depressed patients have cognitive impairment, sometimes referred to as depressive "pseudodementia". Such patients commonly complain of impaired concentration and memory deficits.

Chapter 3

THE ELUSIVE MIND OF MAN

This chapter begins by questioning the relationship between mind, or conscious awareness, on the one hand and the biological functioning of the brain on the other. The relation of brain to mind is beyond question. Contemporary neuroscience has gone far in understanding and unlocking the incredibly complex secrets of the brain, and, as in other advanced research, the unlocking of one door has led to another more intriguing door.

The processes by which brain produces mind are inherently covert and obstinately elusive. Man has thus been free to give full scope to poetic inventiveness in explaining his experimental being. The fact that the brain is the organ of perception and cognition, and the consequences of this fact, have barely begun to penetrate the vast contrivances of speculation.

Still to be answered is that profound question that looms stark and insistent before all humankind: Is mind a mere molecular mechanism or is there in addition a transcendental quality to awareness? Is man's brain only a magnificently subtle computer or does the brain in its relationship with mind act as the interchange between the physical and metaphysical? The philosophical consequences of the new notion that the mind is modulated by hormones may be as great as the medical and scientific consequences. The double-think of modern science—'Molecules shape the body, but electricity shapes the mind'—ends abruptly with the realization that regulatory hormones control both brain and body functions.

The new hormone-based paradigm for the mind acknowledges that electricity does flow from nerve to nerve and can be measured on the surface of the brain or on the membranes of individual nerves. But these superficial signals are little more than dry echoes of deeper molecular events going on with the cell. Scientists now believe that the mind will be best comprehended by focusing on intercellular events, rather than on superficial electrical signals. Although this is a new paradigm, nearly all of the early experiments demonstrate that regulatory hormones join in holistic patterns that may be understood by organs other than the brain. The mechanisms that drive thought are found all over the body and, wherever they live, they function at their highest level by recognizing the molecular patterns of the combination of hormones that modulate thought.

There is a revolution going on now in **molecular biology**. The brave new world will demand that those making scientific decisions have a thorough knowledge of brain endocrinology. That knowledge now rests in the heads of those who live in basic neuroscience laboratories, and there will be no benefits to patients without educational strategies that carry this information into the heads of physicians, administrators etc. What is most important, patients must come to know and believe that a bold aggressive attack on the problems of the mind is not a fanciful fiction but a modern reality.

Molecular approaches to neural coding has taken a new meaning. The essential function of the nervous system is to receive information from the sense organs, integrate it, make a decision and, by acting on effector organs, put out the appropriate behavior. This can be accomplished only if information is converted into a system of signals that can be handled by the neuronal network. This system of signals, the **neural code**, has been the object of intensive study in recent years (particularly more so by George Ungar).

Returning to the idea in the discussion of the molecular code, it should be noted that any lasting modification of synaptic connectivity must involve chemical changes. Whether it consists in actual anatomical growth, increased synthesis of transmitters or receptors, or recognition between pre- and post-synaptic surfaces, it must have an important chemical component. There is increasing evidence that the consolidation of acquired information is associated with characteristic chemical changes, particularly with increased RNA and protein synthesis. There is also suggestive evidence that the chemical changes are essential for efficient information processing because inhibition of RNA and protein synthesis may cause **impairment of learning**.

The observations just mentioned, although compatible with the molecular coding hypothesis, do not actually prove it. The chemical changes may be entirely non-specific, indicating an increased need for synthesizing neuro-transmitters or receptors, reflecting cell growth or simply the increased metabolism of active neural tissue. None of the methods of chemical analysis available today is entirely capable of deciding whether the proteins synthesized in the learning brain are part of a coding system or are devoid of any such significance.

The problem now is identifying the process by which acquired information, represented by the creation of new connections, become **consolidated**, and persists in the brain for long periods of time and often permanently. The idea of a lasting electrical configuration, the "reverberating circuit" of Lorente de No ('38) has been abandoned because disruption of all electrical activity of the brain by hypothermia or electroconvulsive shock fails to abolish consolidated memory traces. Another long favored hypothesis is the actual morphological growth of new synapses between the pathways to be connected (Eccles; '65). Recent research has shown that synapses are complex structures which are unlikely to be formed during the interval sufficient for the consolidation of memory traces.

The present tendency is to explain the fixation of acquired information by a vague concept of **synaptic facilitation**, involving an increase in the synthesis of transmitters or receptors. Hitherto non-functional but anatomically present synapses could undergo "synaptic validation". According to Cragg ('67), out of the estimated 10^{14} synapses of the human brain, only 1% is functional, leaving a considerable number of them available for the acquisition of new information.

Ungar's interpretation of a molecular code of neural information is based, to a large extent, on the principle of **chemospecificity** of neural pathways (first proposed by Sperry in 1963). Careful observations have shown that during embryonic development the neurons destined to become part of the same pathway recognize each other by a mechanism that can only be explained on a chemical basis.

It seems that at the time of birth, before any learning has taken place, the brain is provided with molecular labels for each of the estimated 10^7 neural pathways. The molecular coding of the innate neural channels has suggested that the modifiability of neural connections in the adults is a continuation of developmental processes. The main conclusion that is beginning to emerge from the work of scientists during the last two or three decades is that neural function, like other activities of living systems, is based on **chemical principles**. It draws the energy necessary for its maintenance from the chemical reactions of its metabolism, the switches which turn synapses on and off are chemical, and now it appears that the machinery by which it is programmed and can reprogram itself may also have a molecular basis. Molecular biology has shown that computation can be done on chemical principles as easily as by electronic means.

When discussing the 'chemistry of mind', perhaps the intricate relation between the abstract mind and the physical brain will always remain shrouded in mystery. But, as the marvels of brain organization are unraveled through painstaking research, it is becoming evident that mind and behavior can be profoundly influenced by quite understandable physical and chemical processes. The human brain is jammed with neurons, each a tiny chemical powerhouse. The neurons are in ceaseless activity, generating minute electrical currents which flicker from cell to cell, providing an interconnecting network of fantastic complexity. The cells of the brain that are involved in conscious activity, awareness of self, emotion, and all the functions we associate with mind possess properties of an order different from any other living cells. Whether these properties derive from the sophistication of their cerebral interconnections, from a set of chemical reactors which have so far escaped notice, or from completely unknown sources cannot even by surmised at this stage of our knowledge. But it is becoming evident that the amine pathways (see Chapter V) have a great deal to do with setting the level of activities of these cells and guiding them toward goal-directed tasks. Words such as motivation, drive, feeling, and satisfaction describe the subtleties of the process.

If proper study of mankind is man, we neuroscientists are guilty of many inappropriate studies, as we have carried out a great deal of research on animals. There are mitigating circumstances, of course; the complexity of the human brain, even as an electrochemical machine, is beyond imagination. When fourteen billion elements, each an intricate assembly of chemical and physical components, are congregated in a network of total connectivity, the number and diversity of interactive patterns is greater than all the particles in the universe. In a real and an overwhelming sense, the universe is bounded by the mind of man. This is, of course, to beg the question of brain and mind, but the basic working hypothesis of brain research is that mental phenomena can be defined in terms of brain activity. The sheer size and complexity of the human brain is not the only reason why neuroscientists have been reluctant to approach it. The variation between individuals (which is really another aspect of its complexity) makes traditional techniques inadequate.

CAN THE MIND CONQUER CANCER?
(Happy people rarely get cancer)

There are signs that nowadays conventional medicine is looking beyond chemical and radiation therapy for deeper and more complex reasons for the scourge of modern society.

At present, questions are being asked about the power of the mind over cancer. This is more so because of the excellent results occurring amongst some patients who began a complete change of life-style and took responsibility for their own treatment.

By eliminating unhealthy over-reaction to stress, stopping smoking, putting your diet under the microscope and developing a positive mental attitude, in many cases can make the difference whether you live or die.

As will be explained later in this book, some stress is necessary, but if people learn not to over-react they will not go beyond the stress limits which could lead to several disorders including cancer.

In Melbourne, in the surgery of new-wave psychiatrist (the late) Dr. Ainslie Meares, groups of cancer patients gather for meditation sessions—de-stressing consultations that the doctor says have produced complete regressions in some cases, without any other form of treatment. The key is the patient's immune system, which fails under stress. If you are feeling down and out and depressed, your immunity goes down.

If you have a lower immunity you have a poorer response to fighting disease. Many patients who looked back about two years prior to getting cancer find they were under some unusual stress and reacted with hopelessness.

Studies of women three months after having small tumors removed from their breasts, indicate that the vital factor was "fighting spirit". Women who in some cases just denied they had cancer at all, did twice as well as those who accepted their fate and felt helpless. This latter group in general lacked the fighting spirit and adopted a very *passive* attitude, without wanting to talk about it or disturb other people.

Please see your doctor if you feel this way. If he/she is too busy a longer appointment will be arranged for you to talk to someone who can help you. *There is a growing body of convincing evidence that the mind and cancer are linked.*

What is of importance here is the extent to which a person reacts to psychosocial stresses in the manner described depends on the personality structure i.e. the significance to which he attaches to the events in question. The stresses involved are social incompatibility, social change, urbanization, change of location, difficulty or dissatisfaction with work, dramatic events, crises, the loss of a close friend or relative, grief, despair, depression and loss of hope. Such stresses can of course precipitate many forms of illness. This has been shown to be the case when patients underwent a change of emotional equilibrium and found their life situation unsatisfactory, threatening, strenuous and conflicting, while being unable to change it. Even slight life changes correlated with some deterioration of health in some people while serious changes were associated with illness in almost 80% of individuals who were subjected to stress.

These correlations were investigated particularly with respect to cardiac infarction and **cancer**. If one assumes that a proportion of malignant tumors are triggered by endogenous viruses, lowered immune activity as a sequel to increased adrenocortical function under psychosocial stress could further the growth of malignant cells. The question of whether emotional psychosocial factors play a role in cancer is very old indeed. Even Hippocrates, the father of medicine, considered it. Present day theories concerning the history of cancer patients reveals particularly frequently: the loss of an earlier, important person of reference; the inability to express hostile feelings and emotion; an abnormally strong emotional attachment to one of the parents; sexual disturbances. These results reveal a distinct correlation between psychosocial factors and the occurrence of illness. They confirm that in the case of some diseases it has not only been possible to prove the significance of psychosomatic factors but also to explain essential points regarding the dynamics involved.

It is interesting to note the findings of a survey of over 3,000 Texan patients suffering from either physical or mental handicaps. This revealed that persons suffering from mental illness had a greatly reduced risk of developing cancer; the risk falling progressively the lower their IQ and level of mental functioning. The doctors conducting the survey excluded a number of possible reasons for this relationship, and concluded that the most likely explanation was that patients with gross mental limitations lived in their own sheltered world and were spared the psychological and physical stress which arises from interaction with the environment.

Man's nervous system is awesomely complex. Network of nerve cells, some with fibres several feet long, run throughout the body connecting every distant bit of tissue with the 14 billion nerve cells of the governing brain. Electrical impulses travel along these pathways at speeds from two to 200 miles an hour, leaving across narrow gaps between cells, relaying intelligence to and from the brain.

Man's mind and mental processes have always seemed to him as mysterious and fascinating as the universe itself but investigation of the nature of the mind has become the province of experimental neuroscience only during relatively recent times. The scientific approach has cast much new light on the nature of our mental processes, on the sources of emotional life, and on the various patterns of behavior. As we acquired new knowledge, simple views have been replaced by more and more complicated questions.

Nevertheless, the elusive mind of man has still mysteries of its own. Will all the mysteries disappear when we understand the functioning of the complex anatomical structure and chemistry of the brain? (see Chapter VI). Man still asks, what is the "mind"? Cognitive psychologists are still fascinated by man's inner mental processes. Many are still studying the original problem posed by scientists long ago: how does the mind perceive? Many psychologists, particularly in America, prefer to study behavior, believing that man's actions can be more accurately observed, and are possibly more significant, than what does on inside his head.

Whatever the nature of the mind, there is no doubt that the mechanism through which it works is the nervous system. In Chapter VI, I explain in detail how the chemical imbalance causes disorders of the mind (the broken brain).

Most of man's nerve activity involves circuits leading through billions of cells of the brain, where innumerable interconnections offer many choices in the response made. Unfortunately, the circuits cannot easily be traced in the brain. The elaborate chemistry of the nerve fibres has been studied in detail and a good deal is known about the chemical processes that keep an impulse moving along the path. But there are still questions on how nerve cells convert energy into impulses initially. Perhaps the most challenging of all the unknown is how these electro-chemical impulses can produce such an astonishing variety of effects, ranging from dreaming to reciting a poem to writing a letter.

Psychologists have wrestled with categories for them, such as conscious - versus unconscious - mental activity and voluntary - versus involuntary - motor activity. But nerve activities cannot be isolated in tight compartments. In practice, all of our mental processes are highly integrated with each other . As a result, the very term "conscious" is one of the most difficult psychologists have to define.

Chapter 4

IS STRESS WORTH WORRYING ABOUT?

Stress—real, heart-stopping stress that gets the adrenaline surging—affects people in all kinds of jobs.

Stress has been linked to every ailment from asthma, to heart disease, to ulcers. Yet the latest medical research indicates there is such a thing as good stress, which can be productive, even healthful, and that high level executives are less susceptible to bad stress than are their underlings, who see themselves as powerless.

A survey taken by the Bell Telephone Company showed that workers on the shop floor had twice as many heart attacks as the company's top-flight executives. This is confirmed by actuarial studies which show that the death rate among American company presidents is only 58% of the average for the country's white males. It seems that contrary to popular belief, stress, far from hastening a successful manager to an early demise, actually helps to prolong his life. This is particularly noticeable among American Presidents, many of whom have lived to a venerable age. It has been shown that U.S. Presidents, unless they meet an unnatural death, live longer on average than Vice Presidents, and longer still than unsuccessful candidates for the Presidency.

Chronic stress is triggered *not* by the pressure of decision-making, but by the feeling that one's decisions are useless, that life is overwhelming and beyond personal control.

If people feel a sense of purpose, view change as a challenge and not a threat, and believe they are in control of their lives, they would not be adversely affected by stress.

While everyone still agrees that stress is bad, and needs to be controlled if people are to live happy and fulfilled lives, the assumption that stress alone causes heart and other disorders, is now under challenge.

It is clear, however, that those who do not cope well with pressure have higher stress levels and these people are much more likely to expose themselves to the risk factors which cause chronic disease, including heart disease.

If you feel that you are not coping well with pressure, consult your doctor soon.

A feeling of being 'under stress' is a common complaint people make about their lives. They mean many things—have too many things to do and not enough time to do them; being vaguely worried a lot of the time and yet not knowing exactly why; feeling tense and irritable almost constantly; and generally feeling that things are not quite right. This bad type of stress seems to be a factor in many common diseases. For instance, there appears to be a close link between the way people live today and the rise in heart disease. Stress-prone behavior is thought to contribute to it. As well, amongst other conditions, stress is thought to be related to some mental illnesses, to obesity, and to drug addiction. Learning to deal with stress is an important part of preventing ill health.

ANXIETY AND TRANQUILLIZERS

"We should live in 'day-tight' compartments. Each day we should pull down a mental curtain, shutting out the past, and another curtain shutting out the future so as to live for today, unburdened by remnants of the past or anxieties about the future." Osler.

As mentioned above, anxiety is usually a healthy response to things that threaten your well-being.

It is natural to feel upset if you are short of money or have difficulties in your marriage.If someone close to you dies, it is natural to feel sad and lonely.

Both men and women get stressed and worried at times, for good reasons. But women are twice as likely as men to have tranquillizers prescribed for them. Even without an outside job, looking after children and the home is demanding, tiring and stressful work, with long hours and not much support from other people.

Taking tranquillizers can make you feel much better in the short term when your problems become extreme, or help you sleep in a time of crisis. Taking them for a short time can be useful. But if they are taken for every difficulty that crops up, or for a long time, they can cause problems.

The elderly are particularly vulnerable to over-sedation from benzodiazepine tranquillizers. Disinhibition, combined with memory loss and confusion, may lead patients on low doses of benzodiazepines to commit a variety of antisocial acts, from shoplifting to sexual offences.

Such patients come to rely on the drugs for psychological comfort and suffer *withdrawal symptoms* if they stop the drug. More commonly, the symptoms are those of an anxiety state, with panic attacks, insomnia, tremors, hyperventilation, increased muscle tension and cardiovascular symptoms.

Occasionally, the syndrome may be severe, worse than the condition for which benzodiazepines were originally prescribed, and may be prolonged for many months.

If you want to stop taking the pills, please *don't* stop suddenly but consult your doctor first. It could be dangerous to stop suddenly; you need to reduce the dose *gradually* over a few months.

Ask your doctor to explain your symptoms—what is causing them and how the treatment should help.

Think about changing some aspects of your life. Learn other ways of relaxing—relaxation exercise, biofeedback technique, massage, yoga, meditation or Tai-Chi.

Learn ways of improving your health and sense of well-being, such as getting regular exercise, eating healthy food, cutting down on other drugs like alcohol and caffeine.

Learn to be more confident for example through an assertive training course.

STRESS-RELATED PROBLEMS

You often hear people using the word "stress" as though it means "distress", something unpleasant. It is to be emphasized that as in other diseases, early treatment of stress-related disorders is most effective.

Hiding the symptoms of stress does not get rid of the strain on the body.

The following are some stress warning signals that should not be ignored: fatigue, tension, headaches, aching neck and shoulder muscles, sleep disturbance, sexual problems, frequent low-grade infections, explosive anger in response to minor irritation, increased intake of alcohol etc. Please see your doctor if you feel this way.

A "Stress Test Check List" is shown on the next page, with the most stressful life event (death of spouse) given a value of 100. Change in the number of arguments with a spouse given a value of 35, and a high mortgage given a value of 31. The list reproduced, with minor modifications, from the *Journal of Psychosomatic Research*.

The social environment is at least as stressful as the physical one. Parents and children often disagree about values, acceptable behaviors and use of family resources. Members of the family may hold unrealistic expectations of one another so that when these expectations are not met, members of the family become angry, frustrated and disappointed.

THE TEENAGE SUICIDE EPIDEMIC

A young teenager commits suicide nearly every day. Suicidal behavior of adolescents has been linked to personal experience of loss and to family violence. Suicidal children are more likely to be from families where there are persistently hostile and tense relationships.

There also appears to be a link with alcohol and drug abuse, while sixty percent of suicidal children have a history of being physically abused.

Young girls are more likely to be suicidal than boys, although the boys' attempts are more likely to be lethal. Among boys, losing someone close to them appears to increase the likelihood of a suicide attempt.

The Social Readjustment Rating Scale

Life Event	Mean Value
1. Death of a spouse	100
2. Divorce	73
3. Marital separation from mate	65
4. Detention in jail or other institution	63
5. Death of a close family member	63
6. Major personal injury or illness	53
7. Marriage	50
8. Being fired at work	47
9. Marital reconciliation with mate	45
10. Retirement from work	45
11. Major change in the health or behavior of a family member	44
12. Pregnancy	40
13. Sexual difficulties	39
14. Gaining a new family member (through birth, adoption, oldster moving in, etc.)	39
15. Major business readjustment (merger, reorganization, bankruptcy, etc.)	39
16. Major change in financial state (a lot worse off or a lot better off than usual)	38
17. Death of a close friend	37
18. Change to a different line of work	36
19. Major change in the number of arguments with spouse (either a lot more or a lot less than usual regarding child rearing, personal habits, etc.)	35
20. Taking on a mortgage greater than $10,000 (purchasing a home, business, etc.) [†]	31
21. Foreclosure on a mortgage or loan	30
22. Major change in responsibilities at work (promotion, demotion, lateral transfer)	29
23. Son or daughter leaving home (marriage, attending college, etc.)	29
24. In-law troubles	29
25. Outstanding personal achievement	28
26. Wife beginning or ceasing to work outside the home	26
27. Beginning or ceasing formal schooling	26
28. Major change in living conditions (building a new home, remodeling, deterioration of home or neighborhood)	25
29. Revision of personal habits (dress, manners, associations, etc.)	24
30. Troubles with the boss	23
31. Major change in working hours or conditions	20
32. Change in residence	20
33. Changing to a new school	20
34. Major change in usual type or amount of recreation	19
35. Major change in church activities (a lot more or a lot less than usual)	19
36. Major change in social activities (clubs, dancing, movies, visiting, etc.)	18
37. Taking on a mortgage or loan less than $10,000 (purchasing a car, TV, freezer, etc.)	17
38. Major change in sleeping habits (a lot more or a lot less sleep or change in part of day when asleep)	16
39. Major change in number of family get-togethers (a lot more or a lot less than usual)	15
40. Major change in eating habits (a lot less food intake or very different meal hours or surroundings)	15
41. Vacation	15
42. Christmas	12
43. Minor violations of the law (traffic tickets, jaywalking, disturbing the peace, etc.)	11

* From Holmes T: Life situations, emotions, and disease. J Acad Psychosom Med 19: 747,1978.

† This figure no longer has any relevance in light of inflation; what is significant is the total amount of debts from old sources.

Society should be protecting youth more, particularly by controlling use of firearms.

Depression and vulnerability in our youth require early attention.

Driven by deep despair, teenagers are taking their own lives in record numbers. Can we restore hope for those on the brink and offer them something to live for? Some talk about the feelings of depression that completely overwhelm them, making the idea of "blotting out" their lives seem appealing and logical. The worst thing about this kind of depression is that they are not in control over it. One girl said: "When you get to that point, you just don't care any more". She tried to kill herself four times between the ages of 16 and 20, with overdose, and by cutting and slashing at her wrists. It is a better alternative, she says, and then, noticing the shock she has caused, adds quietly, "I didn't so much want to die. I didn't want to live".

YOU ARE NOT ALONE ...

Depression—the medical name by which this illness is known—is not a good name.

Like many medical terms it has gradually developed as knowledge of the condition has grown, and is now a recognized and accepted term for a collection of symptoms, which may vary greatly from patient to patient.

Some patients, for example, may just feel fatigued, or not able to sleep, perhaps experience vague aches and pains while others suffer deep feelings of gloom and sadness, lose their appetite and are continually anxious about nothing in particular.

As you can imagine, this great variation of symptoms sometimes make it difficult to diagnose depression quickly (you may not even be able to remember when your first symptoms appeared).

However, through training and experience, your doctor has made the first important step in returning you to good health by recognizing the condition.

Now, with your doctor's help, the help of your family and a real effort from yourself, you are on the pathway to recovery.

Two facts that you must appreciate and which may help you over the difficult weeks ahead:

1. You are not alone:

One of the most frightening aspects of depression is the feeling that you alone suffer these symptoms and that "nobody understands" how you feel.

In actual fact, the condition is quite common and, more importantly, its nature and treatment are well understood by your doctor, who will be able to assist you because of their knowledge of how you feel.

If you have any problems affecting your performance of every day tasks, talk them over with your doctor on your next appointment.

2. **Depression is treatable:**

The basic cause of depression is an upset in body chemistry and because of this, it is possible to treat patients with effective medicine.

Your doctor has access to a number of different medications and can select one or more to suit the individual patient.

Do not expect an immediate miracle. Some symptoms may take a few weeks to be relieved. Your family can help over this period by their patience, understanding and encouragement.

One thing you must accept is that you are suffering from an illness just as real as pneumonia or influenza, and that your medicine has been prescribed to make you well. It is not a sign of weakness or lack of "will-power" on your part that makes these medicines necessary.

In actual fact, depression is most common in the busy, energetic, dependable type of person whose reliability makes them prone to the illness, so don't feel guilty at needing chemical agents to make yourself well again.

There are many different ways you can help yourself not to be worried by stress. You will have to work out which one suits you best. Here are some broad ways of handling stress which should be used together:

1. Having useful ways of looking at stressful situations.
2. Learning to relax.
3. Keeping fit through physical activity.
4. See a counselor (Marriage Guidance or community) about any problems you may have, to do with your personal relationships or work situations.

Useful ways of looking at stressful situations

1. Remind yourself that a physical or mental stress is only a strain when you are not handling it properly. The strain is inside you and is your response to the situation. It is not part of the situation itself.

2. Everyone has problems and they are a normal part of life. The best thing

to do is to learn how to deal with them so that they don't upset you too much.

3. Don't make mountains out of molehills. Say your car breaks down in the middle of peak hour traffic or miles from anywhere in the outback. If you tell yourself what a disaster it is, if you wring your hands and w o n - der why awful things always happen to you and not to other people, you will wind up being upset and it will in fact be a disaster. But if you say to yourself that it is a nuisance or a pity but no more than that, you will probably deal with it better, and certainly more easily.

4. It is possible to avoid some stressful situations. You can get up ten minutes earlier to avoid rushing breakfast for running for the bus. Try to organize things at work so that you are not always rushing round chasing the clock. And try to avoid people or activities you find annoying.

5. Don't try to do everything at once. Choose a few important goals, concentrate on them and decide to let some others go by the board until you have time for them. And don't ask too much of yourself. Do the best you can but don't worry if the result is not absolutely perfect.

6. Talk to someone about your bad feelings of stress. Simply talking about a problem is often the first stage of solving it. Friends and life partners can help by listening and possibly giving you a new slant on your worries. If you would rather talk to someone not so directly involved with you, doctors, social workers and community health workers are there to listen and help. You in turn can help friends in the same way if they need it.

7. Live in the present. Don't dwell on the past disasters or what might have been, and don't waste time worrying about the awful things that might happen in the future. There is nothing you can do to change what has happened so there is no point in worrying about it; and the future disaster may never happen. Concentrate on what you want to do here and now.

8. Do not be reluctant to seek medical help if you are worried about your health. There are always people who are willing and able to help whatever the problem—do not be unwilling to benefit from their experience.

LEARNING TO RELAX

Relaxation is a skill which is easy to learn. It can reduce your level of stress and it can make you less likely to become tense and anxious. It allows you to do more with less physical effort and to think more clearly. You will also become more aware of **muscle tension** in your body which you can deliberately relax if you want to. Regular practice of a **relaxation technique** acts to let off energy which builds up in stressful situations—it lets off steam and provides a balance in daily life.

If you have trouble relaxing parts of your body (particularly the muscles of the neck), it often helps to get someone else to massage the area gently while you think about relaxing it. When not saying the word "relax" to yourself, it is best to keep your mind on tranquil thoughts as far removed as possible from your daily life.

An even simpler and frequently effective method, the relaxation response, consists of quietly breathing with the eyes either closed or fixed on your hand or thumb. Let any thoughts float through your mind or away. Don't try to hold them. With each outward breath say "one" or "relax" softly. Continue to do this. The more often you relax, the more easily you can do it. Try to set aside a regular time once or twice each day for about 10-20 minutes relaxation. Yoga, transcendental meditation and biofeedback techniques help some people. You can also seek advice from local health workers about cassette tapes on relaxation to suit you. You have to find out, possibly by trial and error, what works best for you. It is also a fact that if you have regular physical activity, things do not worry you as much. Fit people suffer less from depression than unfit people.

STRESS MANAGEMENT

Just as stress is conceptualized as involving events, their interpretation by individual, and a physiological response, stress management interventions have been components of the stress response. Stress management programs often combine a number of intervention strategies, making it difficult to determine the active ingredient in a given program or for a given individual.

However, research with one class of interventions, those aimed at attenuating the physiological response to a stress by training the individual to relax, has resulted in clear evidence that relaxation training is a useful intervention for stress-related disorders such as ulcers, hypertension, headaches, irritable bowel syndrome, and various anxiety disorders.

In 1973 researchers have found that the human body had its own opiate receptors. The body makes its own natural pain killers. These are morphine-like substances called endorphins and enkephalins. Although the exact role that endorphins play in responding to stress is unclear, a number of studies have suggested they may modulate a person's specific responses to stressful situations.

Exposure to stress has been shown to increase the body's production of endorphins. It has been proposed that the pleasurable effects associated with exercise (the so-called runner's "high") may be a result of endorphin release triggered by exercise. Although the precise role of endorphins is evolving, this topic remains an important and exciting area of research.

Women who respond to stress with hopelessness have an increased incidence of cervical cancer. The inability to cope with stress is associated with an increased chance of a breast biopsy finding a malignancy. Depressed mood has been linked with an increased risk of cancer. Depressed patients have four times as many unpleasant life events as controls (during the previous nine months). People with high stress levels and poor coping mechanisms have a fourfold increase in risk of developing psychiatric symptoms (compared with patients who have low stress and good coping skills). Depression has been correlated with an increase in social stresses.

Chapter 5

THE BIO-MEDICAL REVOLUTION
IN PSYCHIATRY

Psychiatry, a branch of medicine, is responsible for the study, diagnosis, treatment of human behavior. Abnormal behavior may be determined or modified by genetic physicochemical, psychological, and social factors.

Psychiatry applies knowledge from the biological and social sciences, e.g. genetics, pharmacology, and psychology, to the care and treatment of patients suffering from disorders of mental activity and behavior. It emerged as a branch of medicine in the first half of the nineteenth century when some of those kept under social control for the protection of society in workhouses and other institutions were recognized as curable, i.e. susceptible to **moral** treatment, or requiring the firm although therapeutic use of restraint, and as lying therefore within the province of medicine.

Modern day psychiatry emphasizes the humane and compassionate aspects of medicine. This book is dedicated to that humanism which is often lost in technically based modern-day medical practice. In the United States, psychiatry is the only medical school course consistently taught throughout the four years of the curriculum. It is a dramatic reminder to all of medicine of its mission—diagnosis, treatment, and the elimination of pain, suffering, and disease through the treatment of the **whole person.**

Psychiatry was the last speciality to be incorporated into medicine. Although the study of human behavior is as old as recorded history, it was only within the last two hundred years that, as mentioned above, mental disorders were considered within the province of medicine. The history of psychiatry is, at the same time, the history of civilization. As man increased his knowledge of the world around him, he also increased his knowledge of the world within.

The psychiatrist must muster the knowledge and skills not only of objective observation but also of subjective, participant and self observation. His background in natural science has fostered objective observation, but as he learns other types, he finds this differentiation of his role function is necessary for understanding the relationship to his patient and for growth in his capacity for human intimacy. Only then can the general notion of personality and its underlying principles be learned: the genetic and other factors in growth, development, and decline. Their recognition of unconscious and preconscious factors as determinants of behavior; the idea that the personality is integral and indivisible; and recognition that man is a social animal and that the emerging stages of the life cycle reflect coordination between the evolving individual and his social environment.

The roots of psychiatry are somewhat different from the roots of general medicine. The focus of psychiatry has been on the mind and its disorders. Psychiatry is an application of neuroscience to the problems of a particular group of patients. Because of its philosophical and theological origins, psychiatry frequently asked philosophical rather than **biological** questions. For many years, psychiatry was preoccupied with why things occurred and ignored **how** they have occurred. This ignoring of mechanisms and search for meaning helped to obscure, rather than to enhance, the study of the problems of the human mind.

There is a second tradition in psychiatry which was less based on observation and speculation and more on empiricism. This latter tradition has grown and in recent years has become the dominant force in American psychiatry. The former tributaries now carry definite names, such as biological psychiatry, social psychiatry, cultural psychiatry etc. The urgency of the need to merge these tributaries into a single psychiatry is just to be recognized. Psychiatrists, by the nature of the problems possessed by the patients under psychiatric care, are becoming multi-disciplinary and inter-disciplinary in their perspective.

REVOLUTIONARY ADVANCES IN PSYCHIATRY

Revolutionary advances in psychopharmacology over the past quarter of a century have resulted in the development of a more scientific basis for treating mental illness. Such as psychodynamic insights (see Chapter IX, Freud), the psychological side of psychiatry, drug treatment dramatically changed how psychiatry is practiced, upgraded research from the essay to the controlled clinical trial, and altered practices to take into account the understanding of **neurochemical mechanisms** (see Chapter VI), clinical pharmacology (see Chapter XI, Prozac), and solid empirical data.

As has been common in other fields of science, serendipity, as well as careful scientific investigation, has added to the store of knowledge concerning antipsychotic (neuroleptic) drugs: their mechanisms of action, efficiency in the treatment of major mental illness, principles of administration for optimal results, and range of side effects. The introduction of chlorpromazine (Thorazine) was dramatic, and even though it did not produce a permanent cure for schizophrenia, it benefited many patients in a way that no other treatment had before. News of its effectiveness spread rapidly, and within a year or so chlorpromazine was being used worldwide by hundreds of thousands of schizophrenic patients.

The **therapeutic revolution** initiated by chlorpromazine went far beyond its pharmacological effects. Custodial care changed to active treatment, and alternative forms of treatment were encouraged. The clinically significant therapeutic effect produced by antipsychotic drugs made it possible to discharge many patients from long-term custodial facilities. Persons with schizophrenia who otherwise would have been permanent residents of mental hospitals, had their fate profoundly altered. Many were able to remain out of hospital for considerable periods of time and to function adequately in their communities. Others recovered sufficiently to be transferred to nursing homes, 'half-way' houses, or their own homes, even though they functioned only marginally. For patients remaining in the hospital, the facility became a more **humane** place with more adequate staff-patient ratios and active treatment programs.

Natural history on studies done before the introduction of antipsychotics reveal that two out of three patients with schizophrenia spent most of their lives in the State insane asylum. In contrast, it is now estimated that more than 95% of such patients live outside the hospital, even though many continue to have relapses and residual symptoms. The changes resulting from the introduction of antipsychotic drugs have meant a massive reduction in the number of beds occupied by previous hospitalized for schizophrenia.

This profound alteration in the locus of treatment of mental patients is a most convincing proof of the efficiency of **antipsychotic** drugs. In Chapter VI, I shall also explain how the discovery of **antidepressant** drugs have a similarly profound revolutionary effect, more particularly so after the introduction of Prozac. The discovery of chlorpromazine's antipsychotic effects occurred partly, but not entirely by chance. Chlorpromazine was synthesized as an antihistamine and deliberately chosen for investigation in humans because it was a relatively mild sedative. This property led the French anesthesiologist to try it for reducing surgical stress. Then in 1952 it was tried for schizophrenia. The rest is history.

Chapter VI explains in detail the recent discoveries and contribution of biological psychiatry, which will revolutionize the treatment of mental illness during the 1980's and 1990's. It gives accurate information about the recent explosion of knowledge in the **neurosciences** in general and **psychiatry** in particular. This information will be helpful to those who want to find out more about biologically oriented methods for understanding and treating mental illness.

Not all biological treatments are miraculous cures, of course, and it is important that neither doctor nor patient has excessively high expectations. Most medical illnesses can be ameliorated by medications, but very few are eradicated by medication. Penicillin is truly a "miracle cure" that destroys the bacteria causing pneumonia, but for infectious diseases and a few diseases that are treated surgically, most of the illnesses that afflict human beings are improved by doctors but not cured by them. Biological psychiatry promises some help, and often a great deal of help, but it does not guarantee a miraculous cure for every patient.

In one study, 60% of patients who were treated with imipramine for four months relapsed once treatment stopped. The relapse rate dropped to less than 20% if treatment continued for 12 months. The natural history of depression suggested that patients would have, on average, five episodes during their lifetime. In bipolar depression there was an average of 13 episodes. Treatment strategies and patient education would recognize the high rate of recurrences and aim to prevent them.

Chapter 6

CHEMICAL IMBALANCE IN THE BRAIN IS A MAJOR CAUSE OF DEPRESSION

The revolutionary idea that drugs could exert a specific antipsychotic effect led to a search for other **psychoactive** substances with similar antipsychotic properties. Some drugs were discovered empirically or as a result of the clinical investigation of clinically or structurally related compounds. The result of this research has been the discovery and use of a wide variety of substances that are effective in the treatment of schizophrenia and several emotional disorders. All this will also be explained in more detail in most other chapters of this book.

Almost 100 years ago Sigmund Freud said: "Let the biologists go as far as they can and let us go as far as we can—one day the two will meet". For many years after Freud, patients have undertaken years of unsuccessful treatment by a psychoanalyst and behavioral therapists. Along came antidepressant drugs that proved effective for chronically ill patients. There is a virtual revolution occurring in psychiatry with the discovery that emotional disorders respond to specific medications.

In one form or another, that has become the parable of modern psychiatry, a tale told again and again of wonder drugs that seem to alleviate previously intractable problems. As Freud foresaw, biology and psychiatry have met. They have, moreover, embraced, and brought forth a robust new discipline called **biopsychiatry** that strongly emphasizes the *neurological* underpinnings of emotional illness. Even many traditional talk therapists (psychoanalysts) have taken readily enough to prescribing medications like Prozac antidepressant, which give them more options with patients. They emphasize that you can't treat someone who has acute symptoms with free association or the Pop talking cure. But a new look chemical agent may buffer the system so people can begin to work effectively on their symptoms.

On the other hand, some therapists can't help feeling that the trend to neurology threatens their long-held sovereignty over matters of the mind. They see a danger of psychiatrists becoming, in effect, internists, who "manage" emotional illness the way doctors manage their patients: by administering a drug and monitoring its progress, they feel that being internists of the mind would miss the essence of what has been different about psychiatry; some psychiatrists say "we don't just manage brain molecules".

Biopsychiatry advocates seem scarcely inclined to soft-peddle its achievements, or to hide their disdain for conventional psychotherapy. For example, they are hailing the drug Clomipramine as a kind of "on-off switch" for obsessive-compulsive disorders. One fired-up doctor said that his OCD patients "never, ever" have been helped by psychotherapy. This is what most psychoanalysts do with the patient: they talk to them about "toilet training and hostile feelings toward their parents". One day, the doctor asserted, "every disease is going to be seen as a chemical or an electrical disease".

Biopsychiatry tends to incite high expectations in its followers. Says Dr. Paul Wender: "What we are going to find out about the brain is mind-boggling. Every time a new drug is found, another disease disappears, and makes one very curious about what other diseases have a biological basis".

On the other hand, Dr. Shapiro, the editor of the prestigious *American Psychoanalytical Association Journal*, in an editorial a few years ago alerted readers to this recent and forceful "biologization". Shapiro was very plainly miffed by the biostampede. In his 1989 editorial, he said: "Many act as if the modern psychoanalysts should knuckle under to the new biology and trade in his couches for a new brain-imaging apparatus".

Also, many neuropsychiatrists think that researchers are on the verge of chemical attempts to modify character. Also the new drugs would be aimed not so much at patients as at people who are already functioning on a high level, altering for good their internal moods. One neuropsychiatrist said: "I don't see any fundamental technical obstacle to altering personality with drugs. After all, the traits that make up personality are rooted in neurochemicals". Many feel that 50 years from now we may have drugs that can alter personality profiles; things are moving very fast. To some this may appear like pointless parody of something from *Brave New World*. Indeed, for a minority of psychiatrists, the era of the personality pill has already arrived. Hardly a week goes by without a magazine or newspaper telling us about the pharmacopia of the 21th century, replete with pills that will change the personality. At each issue will be questions that strike at the heart of modern psychiatry. Can drugs develop as helpers for serious mental illnesses, such as depression, obsessive-compulsive disorders and anxiety attacks, also benefit people with minor personality disorders— people who have never suffered from depression, say, but have a gloomy outlook, people who have never suffered from anxiety attacks but who are uptight and anxiety prone? If so, where do you draw the line between therapy and enhancement, between medicine and personality engineering?

THE ELECTROCHEMICAL BRAIN

Now we have to consider why medications are sometimes very essential for the treatment of such disorders as severe depression as psychotherapy alone could not be enough. The human brain is often likened to a switchboard or a computer, since all three receive signals and send out messages. Electrochemical signals cause the nervous system to "flash", "blink" and "hum". It is a complex array of "wiring" made up of over 100 billion neurons, interspaced with supportive elements, the glial cells. In order to arrive at a detailed understanding of how the brain works, it is necessary to consider nature and mode operation of the structural components themselves, *the neurons.*

The neuron is the basic unit or cell of the nervous system, and although neurons vary in size and shape, no two being identical, they do show a common functional organization that makes it impossible to describe a typical neuron. Like other cells, the neuron has a plasma membrane, a nucleus and various organ cells within the cytoplasm. It is a single cell and not structurally continuous with any other cell. Extending from the cell body is a single, long fibre-like extension referred to as the axon which ends in a synapse. The synapse is a gap between one cell and another and usually the neurotransmitter is found in that synaptic junction.

The language of the neuron is an electrochemical one. Sometimes it is difficult to comprehend that thoughts, emotions, learning, and myriad functions that are carried by neurons via electric charges known as nerve impulses, but this is indeed the case.

THE SYNAPSE AND NEUROTRANSMITTERS

The junction between one neuron and the next or between neuron and effector is called a synapse and the intervening space is called the synaptic cleft. The synapse has the capacity to transmit some signals and not others, and thus it acts as a gate for a neuronal transmission. A constant interplay between excitatory and inhibitory synapses determines whether a single neuron will fire. All nerve cells use this process to transmit impulses. This process can take place at incredible speeds.

SECRET OF BRAIN CHEMISTRY

While the brain's circuitry remains theoretical, scientists are rapidly revealing the secrets of its chemistry. In recent years, researchers have discovered nearly 40 chemicals that act as neurotransmitters, each designed to convey a different type of information.

Neuromessengers: Neuromessengers is a generic term for neurotransmitters, or neurohormones. Neurotransmitters are the classic neuromessengers that are released rapidly by the pre-synaptic neuron, diffuse across the synaptic cleft, and have either an excitatory or inhibitory effect on a post-synaptic neuron. There are three classes of neurotransmitters—biogenic amines, amino acids, and peptides. The biogenic amines (monoamines) consist of three catecholamines (dopamine, norepinephrine, and epinephrine), and serotonin, and acetylcholine. The biogenic amines account only for 5-10% of the synapses of the human brain, whereas the amino acid neurotransmitters may account for up to 60% of the synapses.

The concepts of supersensitivity and subsensitivity are applied to receptors. These properties signify that a specific neuron is more or less sensitive, respectively, to a constant amount of neurotransmitter.

RESEARCH APPROACHES TO NEUROTRANSMISSION IN NEUROPSYCHIATRY

Assessing neurotransmission in disease states.

The most common approach to assessing neurotransmission status in disease state is to measure one of the following variables: Neurotransmitter synthesizing enzymes, neurotransmitters, or neurotransmitter metalobites. These measures provide a first approximization of neurotransmitter status in the brain. It also is possible to measure neurotransmitter and receptor characteristics in brain tissue post-mortem.

Norepinephrine and Epinephrine: The largest population of noradrenergic neurons are to be found in the brain stem. The axons of these neurons, ascend to the cerebral cortex, limbic system, (including the hypothalamus).

Norepinephrine and Psychotropics: Both the tricyclic antidepressants (TCAs) and the monoamine oxidase inhibitors (MAOIs) affect the limbic system. The acute effect of TCAs is to block reuptake of norepinephrine and serotonin. The acute effect of MAOIs is to block the metabolism of norepinephrine and serotonin. Thus, both antidepressants acutely increase the concentration of these biogenic amines in the synaptic cleft. The acute effects of both antidepressants cause sedation.

Norepinephrine and Mood Disorders: The major hypothesis regarding norepinephrine is the monoamine hypothesis of mood disorders, which states that depression is a result of too little noradrenergic and/or serotonergic activity and this activity is increased by TCAs and MAOIs. There are three major problems with the original hypothesis: 1. There are 3-to-4 weeks' delay between the acute biochemical effects of increasing synaptic norepinephrine and serotonin and the clinical effect of reduced depression. 2. There are drugs that are potent reuptake blockers that are more effective antidepressants; and 3. Newly developed antidepressants that have no reuptake blocking activity of MAOI-like activity are clinically effective as antidepressants. The most recent theory is that the therapeutic effect of all antidepressants is produced by a decrease in the number of postsynaptic β receptors and decreased responsiveness of serotonin receptors. These receptor changes are seen approximately three weeks after initiation of treatment, thereby correlating with the time course of clinical treatment.

SEROTONIN

Serotonergic neurons have their cell bodies in the upper brain stem. These neurons project to the limbic system and cerebral cortex. Serotonin is released into the synaptic cleft upon synaptic stimulation. Once inside the synaptic cleft, serotonin binds to serotonergic receptors. The major mechanisms of deactivation of serotonin is reuptake into the presynaptic terminals.

Serotonin and Psychtropics: Catecholamines and serotonin are interrelated. Antidepressants, for example, affect both noradrenergic and serotonergic synapses. Most tricyclic antidepressants (except desipramine) acutely block **serotonin reuptake** and chronically (after about three weeks) down-regulate postsynaptic serotonin receptors. L-tryptophan affects the serotonin system by supplying more of the amino acid precursor, thereby pushing the pathway to synthesize more serotonin. L-tryptophan has been used both as a hypnotic and as an antidepressant.

Serotonin and Psychopathology: Serotonin has been implicated in mood disorders, anxiety and violence. The acute effect of TCAs and MAOIs to increase the availability of serotonin (and norepinephrine) in the synaptic cleft led to the inclusion of serotonin in the **monoamine hypothesis** of mood disorders. (Ref: Stark, Fuller & Wong; '85)

Acetylcholine: In humans, there is a group of cholinergic neurons in the brain stem that project to the cerebral cortex and limbic system. There is also a group of cholinergic neurons in the nucleus basalis of Meynert that projects to the cerebral cortex and limbic system. These neurons degenerate in Alzheimer's Disease, Down's Syndrome and Parkinson's Disease. Anticholinergic drugs are used to treat the Parkinsonian side-effects of antipsychotic drugs. TCAs block muscarinic receptors thereby causing the side-effects of blurred vision, dry mouth, constipation. ACh has been implicated in the pathophysiology of mood, with an **overactivity of cholingergic** pathway suggested in **depression.**

Acetylcholine and Depression: Acetylocholine (ACh) is involved in sleep, particularly in the production of REM sleep. In animal studies, injection of Cholinergic muscarinic agonists into the reticular formation neurons results in a shift from wakefulness to REM sleep. Disturbance in central cholinergic activity are associated in sleep changes in major depression. As compared to healthy people and psychiatric controls, depressed patients have marked disruption of REM sleep patterns. Administration of a cholinergic agonist, such as arecoline, to depressed patients during the first or second NREM periods results in a rapid onset of REM sleep. It is postulated that depression is associated with an underlying **supersensitivity to ACh.**

Another intriguing observation suggests a link between ACh and depression. Drugs that reduce REM sleep, such as antidepressants, produce beneficial effects in depression. Indeed, about half of the patients with major depression experience temporary improvement when deprived or restricted from sleep. Narcolepsy, which is characterized by both manifestations of REM sleep, is aggravated by compounds that enhance or mimic cholingeric activity. Patients with Alzheimer's Disease have sleep disturbance characterized by reduced REM. Loss of cholinergic neurons in the basal forebrain has been implicated as the cause of these changes.

Chapter 7

DISORDERS OF THE
"LIMBIC SYSTEM" OF THE BRAIN

Analysis of the neuronal organization of the limbic system reveals the very intimate relationship of the amygdala with highly integrative subcortical structures. Fibres from the amygdala converge mainly upon the septum and hypothalamic regions; in addition, impulses from the amygdala reach the hippocampus via the piriform cortex. In turn, the hippocampus discharges into the same septa-hypothalamic zone by way of the fornix. This anatomical arrangement creates favourable conditions for a very close function coordination between the amygdala and the hippocampus. The important role of this anatomical and functional relationship becomes more and more apparent, for it seems evident that the reinforcing effect of such motivational forces as emotion, as well as the laying down of memory traces, are equally essential for the selection of behavioral patterns (see Gloor; '60 and Olds; '58).

The central position of the hypothalamus in emotions depends upon its function as the chief outlet of the neural messages chiefly from primitive parts of the brain to effector organs, striated muscles, smooth muscles and glands. One of the oldest parts of the brain involved in behavior is the reticular formation of the brain stem. This poly-synaptic structure is situated centrally in the midbrain and extends rostrally to the hypothalamus, sub-thalamus and thalamus to affect behavior in a complex fashion. Some reticular impulses are transmitted directly to the neocortex.

Stimulation of the amygdala can produce arousal reactions of many different kinds. These arousal effects are widespread and involve many neuronal systems, both autonomic and somatic. In some ways they are reminiscent of the effects found from stimulation of the midbrain reticular formation. There is ample evidence of differentiation within the amygdala for this behavioral dimension, too. The arousal system of the amygdala seems to be independent of the midbrain reticular formation since the arousal effects produced by amygdala stimulation can be found after lesions of the midbrain reticular formation. The cortical arousal effects initiated from the dorsal amygdala stimulation can suppress epileptiform discharges produced by the application of penicillin to the neocortex.

Clinical observations suggest that the limbic system, unlike the neocortex, derives subjective information in the form of emotional feelings which influence behavior required for self-preservation and the preservation of the species (MacLean; '62). The most important evidence for this is provided by clinical cases with epileptogenic foci in or near the limbic cortex. As Penfold and Jasper ('54) have demonstrated during surgical intervention in such cases, either with the epileptic charge itself or with electrical stimulation of the involved cortex, patients may experience a wide variety of vivid emotional and visceral feelings.

NEURAL SUBSTRATES OF LIMBIC EPILEPSY

The Amygdaloid Connections as a Substrate for Limbic Epilepsy.

It has been shown that of all subcortical areas tested, the amygdala has one of the lowest thresholds for EEG seizures and overt convulsions following electrical stimulation (Alonso-de Florida and Delgado; '58; Delgado et al.; '71; Goddard et al.; '69). The ictal symptoms of temporal lobe epilepsy are well known since the days of Hughlings Jackson (1899) who described them in detail under the heading "Uncinate Group of Seizures". Jackson described aural automatism occurring in uncinate fits as licking, chewing, tasting, and smacking movements. In the opinion of Magnus et al., ('52), masticatory seizures involve a disturbance of consciousness and constitute a type of automatism. Salivation, taste, and smell may be ictal accompaniments, suggesting that the area from which masticatory seizures originate is a sensorimotor region for oral functions. These authors concluded that, to obtain mastication from the temporal region, a subcortical mechanism must be activated, and the most likely subcortical structure is the amygdala.

As mentioned above, some clinical features of certain temporal lobe epilepsy probably reflect amygdaloid functions within the lower range threshold and outbursts of aggression suggest an upset in the function of the amygdala. Following such seizures, aggressive behavior may occur in individual cases as part of a confusion state. The interictal features of temporal lobe epilepsy such as sudden or violent outbursts of rage and irritability can possible be understood in terms of the amygdala. The limbic system appears to play an important part in the experience of fear and anger and in initiating the associated patterns of behavior. Egger and Flynn ('63; '67) stress the fact that one of its important functions, and of the amygdala in particular, is to modulate the activity of other areas, especially the hypothalamus. The limbic system receives signals from cortical and other centres concerned with the external environment and other signals indicating the internal environment. It is suitably placed to compute requirements and to initiate appropriate actions which will be subject to modification by previous learning experiences and, particularly in man, through the intervention of the frontal cordorsomedial nucleus of the thalamus (MacLean; '58) which permit predictions of the possible outcome of the proposed course of action. Kluver and Bucy ('37) described the effects of bilateral temporal lobectomy on rhesus monkeys. Of the various components of the Kluver/Bucy syndrome the most obvious is tameness and placidity which can be regarded as an unresponsiveness to fear and anger-provoking stimuli. Lesions restricted to the amygdala have a similar effect and have been demonstrated in a wide range of animals (Goddard; '64). Amygdalectomized animals can still show normal aggression and fighting if the stimulus is strong enough.

Chatrian and Capmann ('60) could, by stimulation of the amygdala, provoke all the EEG characteristics of psychomotor fit, but this would not occur upon isolated stimulation of the hippocampus. They never found any seizure activity on the cortical electrodes without activity in the amygdala, but amygdala activity was frequently found in paroxysms without any reflection of this on the cortical electrodes. Stimulation of the amygdala can produce arousal reactions of many different kinds. These arousal effects are widespread and involve many neuronal systems, both autonomic and somatic. In some ways they are reminiscent of the effects found from stimulation of the midbrain reticular formation.

Synergy of Mesolimbic Cholinergic-Monoaminergic Mechanisms.

The cell bodies of monoaminergic (MA) neurons occupy different situations in the brain from those of cholinergic neurons, but the course and distribution of their fibres are to some extent similar. Both are largely a heavy cholinergic and DA innervation. The two systems operate in close synergy. Dopamine in particular has been implicated as an inhibitory transmitter in the amygdala (Ben-Ari et al.; '77). The apparent presence of *cholinergic* and *monoaminergic* neurons in the limbic system suggest a certain parallel with the peripheral autonomic nervous system. In the hippocampus, for example, histo-chemical stains have indicated that its main afferent pathways are cholinergic in type. On the other hand, radioautographic and fluorescent studies have detected a notable concentration of NA in the hippocampus. Serotonin studies have indicated a relatively high concentration in the grey matter of the hippocampus.

These findings are of special interest in view of the evidence that tranquil-izing and psychotropic drugs known to affect the metabolism of serotonin and noradrenaline appear to have some predilection of action on hippocampal function as revealed by changes in the EEG (MacLean; '70). MacLean also points out that the limbic system seems not only to exert powerful influences on the autonomic and neuroendocrine centres, but may also be the reacting organ to double antagonistic (and probably synergistic) innervation of the peripheral organs. Finally, there is a difference between the central cholinergic and MA systems that recalls a distinction between the parasympathetic and sympathetic innervation of the periphery, and which may well have functional implications: the cell bodies of MA neurons tend to be further removed from their target areas. In some regions of the brain e.g. the superior colliculus and the olfactory tubercle, and also the neostratum, the cholinergic innervation appears to be largely an intrinsic one. This suggests that the MA systems are more divergent than the cholinergic systems and may be expected to produce more generalized effects.

LIMBIC EPILEPSY AND THE DYSCONTROL SYNDROME

Descriptive associations between limbic epilepsy and mental disorders are very old and are found throughout the literature. Recent investigations have shown that dysfunction of the limbic system of the brain underlies many disturbances of emotion and may result in some psychotic manifestations. The interseizure symptomatology of some patients with psychomotor (limbic) epilepsy may be indistinguishable from that of paranoid schizophrenia. Irritative lesions in or near the limbic cortex give rise to epileptic discharges accompanied by emotional feelings of terror, fear, strangeness, unreality, sadness, wanting to be alone, and feelings of paranoid nature (MacLean; '70). There may be also distortions of perception, again reminding one of the endogenous toxic psychosis. MacLean believes that of all the clinical entities there is perhaps none that has a greater potentiality for shedding light on mechanisms underlying psychic functions in man than psychomotor or limbic epilepsy.

Ervin et al. ('55) found that 81% of 42 patients with EEG foci in the temporal lobes had a diagnosis of schizophrenia, whether or not there was an associated epilepsy. Personality disorder is the most frequent diagnosis. Depression is next, followed by the diagnosis of inadequate personality and psychosis. In both men and women who continued to have psychiatric symptoms, delusions were much less prominent than depression. Reports have also been made of patients with schizophrenia-like psychosis. Thought disorder and blunt affect, as well as primary delusions and hallucinations, were present, and occasionally, catatonic features. The criteria for defining aggressive behavior were acts of explicit physical violence. Most of the aggressive patients were young boys with an early age of onset of seizures.

In recent years there has been increased recognition of the occurrence of seizures involving behavioral automatisms. Visceral disturbances and personality and thought disorders (Baldwin and Bailey; '58; Gastaut, '53; Glaser and Dixon; '57; Glaser, '67; Lennox, '60; Penfield and Jasper, '54). They appear in at least 25% of all seizures states in childhood and in over 50% of those in adult life. They may co-exist with generalized and grand mal convulsions, but occur much less frequently in association with petit mal epilepsy. This complex seizure disorder has been designated as "psychomotor" because of its common association with lesions of the temporal lobe and its involvement with temporal lobe functions, the term "temporal lobe seizure" has also been applied, particularly since the investigations of Jackson ('31). However, the disturbances of functions involved in these seizures strongly implicate the integrated structures considered to be within the *limbic lobe,* and in 1953 Fulton suggested that these be regarded as "seizures involving the limbic lobe".

Pathological Substrates of Limbic Epilepsy.

The pathological changes underlying temporal lobe epilepsy and their pathogenesis have been considered by several groups of neuroscientists working in this field. Analysis of the pathological findings show that small focal lesions were encountered in about 25% of the cases; the location of such lesions was found to be particularly marked in the anterior, inferior, and inferomedial portions of the temporal lobe. In the remaining cases diffuse and disseminated lesions comprising cortical atrophy and white matter gliosis in varying proportions were observed ranging from marked to minimal. In some of the more severely affected cases sclerosis of the hippocampus (Ammon's horn) usually extending to the uncus was also observed, and less frequently of the amygdala as well (Falconer et al.; '58).

It has been shown that in cases with diffuse lesions there is a more frequent history of epilepsy, a higher incidence of abnormal birth, a younger age of onset of epilepsy, and a frequent association of hemiatrophy of the skull, all indicating that frequently the epilepsy arose in early childhood. When the variety of personality disorders were compared with the pathological findings, certain important distinctions could be discerned. Thus in the subgroup of cases with Ammon's horn sclerosis outbursts of aggressive behavior were noted in more than half the cases, a proportion nearly twice as great as in any other subgroup. Grand mal was present in only a few of the tumors and haematomas, while it was present in more than half the cases with diffuse lesions.

Certain fit characteristics were analyzed for their incidence in the main subgroups without any striking correlations being noted. The incidence of abdominal, cephalic, olfactory and gustatory, fear, familiarity, strangeness, memory, and *déjà vu* sensations was approximately the same throughout the various subgroups, as was the incidence of mastication during seizures. The commonest aura by far in the two groups was an abdominal (usually epigastric) sensation. These observations are in keeping with the dictum that is not so much the nature of a pathological process which determines the fit-pattern as its site.

There is also a marked similarity in the EEG findings of the various pathological subgroups. It is noteworthy that in almost half the cases with tumor or haematoma, lesions which presumably are strictly unilateral in situation, there was an apparently independent subsidiary focus of spike discharges in the opposite temporal lobe. It is also noteworthy that independent subsidiary foci in the opposite temporal lobe were also noted in a similar proportion of the cases with disseminated lesions (with or without Ammon's horn sclerosis). However, if a showing spread of discharges from the ipsilateral temporal lobe to the opposite temporal lobe were also included, the proportion in which the opposite temporal lobe was involved was greater with Ammon's horn sclerosis than in the other subgroups.

Scrutiny of the various operative results suggest that there are certain diagnostic criteria by which one can tend to predict the underlying pathology, and so anticipate the therapeutic result. Thus in the subgroup of focal discrete lesions was usually found an onset of epilepsy in adult life, no family history of epilepsy, absence of a history of abnormal birth or infantile epilepsy, symmetry of the skull, and with air encephalograms perhaps another diagnostic or a relative smallness of the temporal horn. In spite of the tumorous nature of many of the lesions, symptoms may have been present for many years (a mean of 10 years in some cases). Falconer, et al. ('58) emphasized that if there is a personality change, a history of aggressiveness is often present. With this background and no other obvious etiological factor such as severe head injury or arteriosclerosis apparent in the history, the likelihood of a tiny tumor or of a haematoma must be considered.

The Kindling Model of Limbic Epilepsy.

Adamec ('80) presented evidence on lasting behavioral after effects of repeated amygdaloid stimulation. Adamec's data show that predatory behavior in the cat can be altered following daily repeated amygdaloid stimulation. He did not stimulate his cats to the point of behavioral convulsions, but repeated the stimulus a few times to lower the after-discharge threshold. This was done bilaterally. The rat killing behavior of these cats was studied before and after the threshold reduction. Several other studies on the kindling effects were reported recently by Racine et al. ('76). Of central importance to the present argument (kindling model of limbic epilepsy) are the data of these investigators showing marked alteration of evoked potentials following kindling in the amygdala. Potentials evoked in secondary sites by test pulses applied to the primary (kindled) focus are increased in amplitude following kindling. All components of potentials evoked in the hippocampus, preoptic area, ventromedial nucleus of the hypothalamus and frontal pole by amygdaloid stimulation were increased in amplitude following amygdaloid kindling.

If changes in synaptic transmission underlie the kindling phenomenon, and if these changes may also underlie other more normal physiological processes (e.g. learning), then it is important to consider the pattern of activation required to produce these changes. Racine and colleague determined that it was necessary to trigger epileptiform discharges in order to develop most of the kindling effects. Stimulation that was below after-discharge did not appear to facilitate subsequent kindling with suprathreshold stimulation. If after-discharge were required to produce the kindling effects then it was felt it was necessary to determine the pattern of cell discharge which occurred during an afterdischarge. The authors found that the afterdischarge-mimicking pattern of stimulation produced a very strong recruiting response in secondary sites when applied to the amygdala and was effective in the triggering of "first trial" generalized convulsions if run continuously for several minutes.

If one may generalize from the stimulation pattern back to the after-discharge pattern on which it was based, then one of the striking features of an epileptiform discharge is that it is ideally suited for the production of a strong potentiation effect on secondary foci. It seems a likely possibility that the potentiation characteristics of amygdaloid after-discharges might be critical to the kindling phenomenon.

Most of this work has been done on amygdaloid kindling, which probably serves as a good model for most *limbic kindling*. Although the kindling effect can be obtained from stimulation of areas outside of the amygdala, responsive areas are largely restricted to the limbic system and related structures. Within the limbic system, the amygdala has been found to be particularly responsive. There is also a suggestion that the responsiveness of particular areas is related directly to the extent of their connections with the amygdala. Limbic system epileptiform after discharge develop as the experiment progresses.

Several experiments have shown that the changes in neural response underlying many of these developments are not restricted to the primary (stimulated focus). After completion of amygdaloid kindling, for example, fewer stimulations are required in secondary limbic sites to develop generalized seizures, even after removal of the "kindled" primary focus. These "transfer" experiments established that transnaptic changes in neural response were developing as a result of the kindling treatment. There are a number of features of the kindling effect which are consistent with the hypothesis that synaptic transmission is permanently facilitated between neural structures as a result of kindling. It has not yet been determined, however, that the kindling effect is a result of changes at the synaptic level. Nevertheless, in view of the fact that many examples of synaptic plasticity have been demonstrated, it seems reasonable at this stage to concentrate on the synapse and in neurotransmitters in our investigation of the kindling phenomenon.

LIMBIC CHOLINERGIC HYPERSENSITIVITY

It was explained above that there are some data which supports the hypothesis that synaptic transmission is permanently facilitated between neural structures as a result of the kindling effect. We will now concentrate on the possible neurotransmitter mechanisms underlying limbic epilepsy. The changes in neural response underlying the kindling processes are not restricted to the primary focus. After completion of the amygdaloid kindling, fewer stimulations are required in secondary limbic sites to develop seizures, even after removal of the kindled primary focus. These "transfer" experiments established that trans-synaptic changes in neural response were developing as a result of the kindling process. Several lines of evidence demonstrate that when the amygdala is stimulated, either electrically or chemically, long-lasting changes occur somewhere in the limbic brain. These changes may be irreversible. The effect can be related to seizure activity present at the time of stimulation.

Participation of Muscarinic Cholinergic Receptors in Kindling.

During recent years there has been increasing evidence of the involvement of cholinergic mechanisms in the cortical mediation of desynchronized activation of the EEG which characterizes the "arousal" response. Celesia and Jasper ('66) have shown that the rate of liberation of acetylcholine (ACh) from the surface of the neostigmized cortex in the cat may increase two to four times during desynchronized cortical activations with arousal, as compared to that obtained during slow wave and spindle sleep. Furthermore, studies of chronically isolated cortex, which have been reported to show spontaneous epileptiform discharges, show increased sensitivity to topically applied ACh (Echlin and Battista; '63) . Increased reactivity of the isolated cortex to ACh suggests that supersensitivity to endogenous ACh may be a factor in cortical epileptogenesis.

Partial or total isolation of the cerebral cortex was offered recently as a model for the study of focal epilepsy but several investigators (see Ferguson and Jasper; '71; Chu et al.; '71; Spehlmann, et al.; '71). These authors investigated the implications of denervation (or "disuse") superdensitivity to putative transmitters. Echlin and Battista ('63) indicated that after weeks or months, the isolated cortex showed spontaneous epileptiform discharges and increased sensitivity to topically applied ACh. Isolated cortex may sustain prolonged epileptiform afterdischarges. This is one measure of supersensitivity.

A causal relationship between supersensitivity and an alteration in the cholinergic system has been suggested (Echlin and Battista; '62), based on the observations that there is a decrease in the AChE activity in isolated cortex Hebb et al.; '63 ; Rosenberg and Echlin; '68) and a *decrease in AchE activity parallels the increase supersensitivity*. Increased reactivity of the isolated cortex to ACh suggests that supersensitivity to endogenous ACh may be a factor in cortical epileptogenesis. All my histochemical studies in mammalian brains (referred to above) point to the fact that some of the highest (AChE) activity in the whole brain is to be found in limbic structures, particularly the basal amygdala.

Recently, Chu et al. ('71) studied the effect of cortical undercutting and long-term electrical stimulation on synaptic AChE. These authors found that a *decrease in AChE activity parallels the increase in supersensitivity*. In this investigation the authors were studying partial or total isolation of the cerebral cortex as a model for focal epilepsy. They reached the conclusion that a decrease in the activity of AChE and the supersensitivity in undercut cortex are likely to be the consequences of the loss of cholinergic innervation and of synaptic "disuse" following denervation.

It has been suggested that the phenomenon of supersensitivity of the neuronally isolated cortex may be explained by an increased sensitivity of subsynaptic and possibly nonsynaptic membranes as a consequence of denervation. This is analogous to the supersensitivity observed in denervated muscle. Cannon ('39) suggested that abnormality of cortical cells in epilepsy might be the result of loss of innervation of cells another example of increased sensitivity in denervated structures. The increase excitability has been likened to the degeneration supersensitivity which develops in peripheral structures after interruption of their neural input (Cannon and Rosenblueth; '49).

It is not yet clear if the neural changes that underlay amygdaloid kindling take place within cholinergic circuits or if these circuits simply play a supportive role in seizure development. The possibility that cholinergic circuits are involved in the kindling process is indicated by the fact that atropine retards amygdaloid kindling (Arnold et al.; '73). This and other aspects of cholinergic hypersensitivity have recently been discussed by Burchfiel et al. ('79) who found that ACh was the only neurotransmitter for which they could demonstrate a relationship to kindling phenomena. Vosu and Wise found that repeated cholinergic stimulation (carbachol) produced behavioral seizures after several applications, similar to those seen with electrical stimulation, suggesting an important role for cholinergic circuitry in subcortical propagation of epileptiform activity. Similar results were presented by Wasterlain et al. ('78) who further showed that mixing the injected carbachol with the muscarinic cholinergic antagonist atropine reduced seizure. It has recently been reported (Girgis; '80) that only a few electrical kindling stimuli are needed to produce prolonged supersensitivity to intracerebrally injected physostigmine. This supersensitivity is correlated with further progression of kindling. Scopolamine, given I.M, in doses of 120 ug/kg, suppresses this kindling induced seizures.

Our own findings and those mentioned above show that cholinergic kindling sensitivity of limbic structures parallel electrical kindling sensitivity (Girgis; '80). This fits best with the hypothesis that it is cholinergic circuits at the site of stimulation that mediate both *electrically* and *chemically* induced kindling (Girgis; '81) and that are involved in the retardation of seizure development by anticholinergic drugs. McNamara ('78) found a selective, transient reduction in muscarinic cholinergic receptor binding in both the stimulated and centralateral amygdaloid regions following kindling. Engel and Sharpless ('77) performed a study to examine the hypothesis that kindling itself might produce a decrease in catecholamine-mediated inhibitory influences of the stimulation site, since this could be one mechanism of kindled alterations in excitability. As indicated earlier in this chapter, dopamine in particular has been implicated as an inhibitory transmitter in the amygdala. The data reported by Engel and Sharpless mentioned above are consistent with the hypothesis that the enduring focal hyperexcitability produced by kindling stimulation may, in part, be attributed to an enduring stimulus induced focal decrement in the catecholmediated inhibition at the site of stimulation.

A permanent alteration in neuronal excitability probably underlies the human epileptic state, particularly the post-traumatic epilepsy, which is most likely to be related to kindling. Some patients who seem to have made good recovery from head injury become epileptic at some time later. Penfield ('56) indicated, that an "incubation" period elapses between the causative brain trauma and the first epileptic attack, and the underlying process may require months or even years to reach fruition. The fact that scopolamine significantly suppressed the kindling-induced seizures in our experiments could have implications for the pharmacological therapy of epilepsy (Girgis; '81).

THE USE OF GLUTAMATE AND KAINIC ACID IN LIMBIC RESEARCH

During the last few years, the use of kainic acid (KA) proved to be a useful tool for investigating metabolic and pathological changes in epilepsy (Tremblay et al.; '83). These investigators described an increased glucose uptake in a number of cerebral structures following intra-amygdaloid injections of KA. Most of these structures belong to, or are closely related to, what is traditionally called the "limbic system". The structures that show an increased glucose consumption, subsequent to KA injections are, with few exceptions, identical to those that are sensitive to the toxic effect that KA exerts on structures distant to the site of injection.

Using kainic acid (either alone or combined with glutamic acid), we have studied its epileptogenic properties and also the associated degenerative changes occurring in limbic structures (Girgis; '85). The prolonged depolarizing effect, with subsequent lowering of threshold of stimulation that would be associated with an abnormal accumulation of excessive quantities of glutamate, we have been able to successfully chemically kindle the amygdala obtaining stage 4 seizure. Intracerebral implantation of 'chemitrodes' was done in limbic structures of cat brain. In some experiments, repeated injections were made by a microsyringe. In others, steady-state flow of glutamate was produced by means of an osmotic minipump, lasting one to two weeks.

In some experiments, we used KA in minimal doses prior to the glutamate minimum, and this catalyzing the reactor, acted as a primer in the production of the original (pathological) locus as found in the human disorder. Stage 6 seizure was observed in these preparations. In these preparations, the pathological changes in the uncus and CA3 fields of the hippocampus correspond well with the metabolic changes as studied by the deoxyglucose method of Tremblay et al., ('83) mentioned above. The present study indicates that intense amygdaloid epileptiform discharge plays a role in the pathogenesis of remote lesions. It is also likely that these excitotoxins have a role in the brain damage associated with sustained limbic seizures.

Recent studies support the theory of glutamate as an endogenous neurotoxin and is therefore capable, via its necrotizing effect, of producing the epileptic focus associated with limbic epilepsy.

GENERAL DISCUSSION AND CONCLUSIONS

The main object of this work has been to describe the implication of the limbic system in psychiatric disorders. The *limbic system,* which has now assumed a conspicuous importance in brain research, is comprised of the great *limbic lobe of Broca* and its subcortical cell stations (amygdala, septum, hypothalamus, thalamus, and reticular formation). The limbic system influences many phases of autonomic function as well as patterns of emotional behavior. It also serves to integrate the higher intellectual functions of the neocortex with the more primitive visceral functions. The results of experimental studies of the present author on the limbic system and particularly in relation to emotional changes has been described and discussed. In spite of the extensive neurophysiological, neuroanatomical and clinical data that have accumulated in recent years, the functional significance of some parts of the structures included in the limbic system is not yet clear. The major portion of *Papez's* hypothesis concerning emotional behavior has gained fairly adequate experimental support. However, it should be pointed out that most of the experimental data have confined parts of the limbic system which influence autonomic activities to a rather limited portion of its rostral part. This comprises the amygdala, frontotemporal polar region, anterior cingulate gyrus, septum and hypothalamus, parts which lie close within what Pribram and Kruger ('54) have called the "second system" of the rhinencephalon. The posterior portion of the cingulate and hippocampal gyri or the hippocampus-fornix system, parts which lie close within the "third system" of Pribram and Kluver, appears to be more concerned in the higher 'psychic' functions rather than in physiological activities of a primitive elementary type. Data are at present accumulating which tend to show that the hippocampal-cingulate system might possibly be critically concerned in memory function (Jasper, Gloor and Milner; '56).

It is reasonable to suppose that of all limbic structures the *hippocampus* represents perhaps the highest level of integration. It is clearly established that it is an important relationship with the reticular activating system and it is very likely that it modifies its activity. Finally it can be said that one cannot exclude the possibility that some parts of the hippocampal-cingulate system are involved in perception, integration or expression of emotional changes. There is clearly much more to be done before we can make a precise and conclusive statement concerning the function of this "third system". But recent work, chiefly by relieving the structures in question of the incubus of olfaction, has opened up a field in which important advances are being made.

To recapitulate, one can say that *Klüver and Bucy's* classical article on bilateral temporal lobectomy which appeared in 1937, and the almost simultaneous paper of Papez on "emotional behavior" have been the stimulus for an unprecedented interest in the *neurological basis of behavior*. Although some portions of the hypothesis of Papez have not gained adequate experimental support, the fiber connections between the various structures concerned are nevertheless a fact and their possible function as an emotional circuit appears to have more validity. The rich variety of autonomic and somatomotor responses evoked from the frontotemporal cortex and the amygdala are all independent of the hippocampus-fornix system. Both the hippocampus and the amygdala, however, are connected with the hypothalamus and thus connected via the thalamus with the cingulate cortex. There are almost certainly two-way connections. One can therefore postulate that in primitive animals the amygdala and hippocampus control the *emotional drive* with whose execution the hypothalamus is concerned. With the development of the cingulate gyrus the control shifts to a higher level. The reason why the limbic system has now assumed such conspicuous importance lies in the fact that it may serve to integrate the higher intellectual functions of the neocortex with the more primitive visceral functions.

MacLean ('52), who has elaborated the theory of Papez, maintained that the limbic lobe of Broca and its subcortical cell stations form a system which is concerned with a variety of emotional and visceromatic reactions, and he named it the "limbic system". All of the recent experimental neuroanatomical and neurophysiological data are in favor of MacLean's concept.

From the foregoing account and discussion one can see rather clearly the implication of the limbic system in psychosomatic disorders. The importance of the emotions in apparently purely physical ailments has already been mentioned under the heading, Psychosomatic medicine. Almost the whole body responds to the discriminating influences of the autonomic nervous system. The nature of the somatic response of each organ in preparation for "fight or flight" is highly specific. The fact that emotional stimuli alone, in the absence of real danger, can produce the same autonomic response patterns suggests that one pathway at least leads to the substrate of emotional activity. The complex nature of the sympathetic response to the awareness of danger indicates the existence of some important integrating center.

The *hypothalamus* is a very important site for the interaction between emotional and somatic spheres. Recent research has also revealed that coordination of arousal responses is mediated by the reticular formation in the brain stem. Here sensory somatic stimuli are received and retransmitted in a diffuse pattern of autonomic, emotional, spinal and cortical arousal. Hypothalamic centers are linked directly with different limbic structures, and via the medial forebrain bundle the limbic system also received impulses from the reticular formation. These stimuli are transmitted and modified by each in turn of the structures comprising the Papez reverberating circuit within the limbic system, each being linked with the others and with neighboring areas of the brain. The resulting interactions make up the complex emotional and autonomic responses to a single stimulus. The original stimulus may be of spinal (sensory) or of cortical (intellectual) origin. The ability of reacting to purely emotional stimuli may acquire *pathophysiological* significance. Whereas the mobilization of the bodily activities to meet an external threat or requirement is obviously vital to survival in emergencies, it is equally obviously unnecessary and even detrimental in the absence of adequate causes (Himwich et al.; '62).

There is also the relevance of the neuroanatomical and functional organization of the limbic system to the tendency of psychosomatic patients to show a confused appreciation of what is happening in the world without and within themselves. In this respect, they are like children or primitive people. "In psychosomatic disorders a confusion manifests itself in multiplicity of ways, whereby disturbances in the external world, are symbolically internalized and given expression through activities of the gut or viscera" (MacLean; '54). In this way the disturbance is expressed on a primitive visceral level, rather than at the higher level of organized thought and action. An individual who feels lonely, rejected and unloved may resort to eating, not only because eating is pleasurable, but because it gratifies his frustrated love needs. This is a good example of a primitive type of confusion that allows person and food to become interchangeable. It is important to keep in mind that overeating and obesity are defense symptoms; they are needed to help the patient in his precarious adjustment to life.

Conrad ('62) emphasized that obesity may be a very complicated psychosomatic problem. Obesity is a result primarily of chronic overeating and, in most instances, overeating is a symptom which is directly related to the emotions. Almost every obese person, if he can be honest with himself, will admit that often he overeats when he feels tense, nervous, unhappy, insecure, lonely, frustrated, etc. And, conversely, if he is happy, relaxed, secure, etc. he has less need to overeat. Thus because of the emotions people may overeat, which if done persistently will result in obesity.

Finally, it remains to say that the so-called "psychosomatic mechanism" is not altogether clear. It is not absolutely well known just how mental conflicts with its resultant anxiety and tension are somehow transmitted to the regulatory centers of somatic function with resultant psychosomatic dysfunction. However, the implications of the limbic system in psychosomatic disorders have been discussed fully.

Psychological upset may sometimes antedate and cause functional impairment, which in turn, may progress to pathologic changes in the cells. As yet we do not understand the functioning of our brain as it receives, retains and later reactivates impulses transmitted to it from the environment through receptor organs, such as the eye and ear. However, these external impulses unquestionably result in a more or less permanent functional alteration in the cellular structures within the brain. To what extent internally originating nervous impulses reaching somatic cells can alter the latter is not altogether completely known.

Significance of the Present Study: It has been estimated that one-third of the general practitioners case-load, excluding psychotics, will consist of persons in whom no organic pathological change can be found to account for the illnesses. Another one-third will have symptoms that are not explained by, or are out of proportion to, any organic disease discovered. Thus, in two-thirds of his patients, the physician must take into account and rectify the mechanism hereby psychic tension finds bodily expression.

In *conclusion* it will be most appropriate to refer to the following statement by Hammett ('62): "When psychiatrists and medical men really develop the field of psychosomatic medicine in all of its ramifications, they will make some of the most dramatic and far-reaching advances toward the relief of human suffering in the history of medicine." We believe that further detailed experimental investigations of the limbic system of the brain will no doubt help greatly towards the fulfillment of this goal.

SCIENTIFIC BASIS OF DRUG THERAPY IN PSYCHOSOMATIC DISORDERS

The history of medicine is full of instances of empirical treatments which were used for many years before their scientific basis became established. There is always a time lag between clinical experience of the effectiveness of a method of treatment and the discovery of its scientific basis. Basic research has helped our understanding of the mode of action of various psycho-active drugs. During recent years, methods have been devised for measuring certain types of brain activity and such information has made it possible to speculate in some detail on the physiologic substrate of emotional activity.

The results of research conducted on the *limbic system* and its role in determining emotional response and controlling the autonomic nervous system was recognized relatively recently. Previously unknown neural circuits have been localized, and this has greatly contributed to our understanding of certain functional relationships. The relevance of these discoveries to actual *therapy* should be obvious, since more detailed knowledge of the function of the various cerebral structures facilitates in more precise localization of the *target area* of psychotropic drugs. The new anti-anxiety drugs will be considered within the coordinates of the neuroanatomical, neurophysiological and pharmacological analysis of their influences on the brain. Himwich ('65) pointed out that it is advisable to use the term "neuropharmacological" when the most apparent action of a drug is on neurological structures, an example of which would be the anti-Parkinson drugs, and "psychopharmacological" where a drug is administered, for example, to allay anxiety or ameliorate psychotic symptoms, but this dichotomous use of the two terms is only a pragmatic device. It is difficult to separate the brain and the mind from each other in the conception which will hereafter be described. Moreover, relations have been uncovered between the extrapyramidal apparatus and mental symptoms. To describe this global action Himwich employed the term "neuro-psychopharmacology", which has come into general use.

Sites of Action of Drugs on the Limbic System: Because every drug affects to a greater or lesser degree all bodily and brain components, it would be surprising if the psychoactive agents did not have many actions throughout the body, but as it turns out, the brain and particularly the limbic system presents sites exquisitely sensitive to these drugs. Usually several limbic structures react in a variety of ways. Thus the emotional components of behavior are influenced most deeply by this group of drugs. The analyses of the areas sensitive to psychoactive drugs were made by Himwich and others on the basis of animal experimentation, though differences of a species are important considerations. It is not suggested that the brain changes disclosed in animals can necessarily be interpreted in such a way that they have significance in relation to behavioral alterations of patients.

Following Domino ('62), a "profile" can be established for each drug based on its effects on the cortex, thalamus, hypothalamus, limbic cortex and brain stem reticular formation. In an analysis of the sites of action of the minor tranquilizers, Himwich described that they exert only weak or no effects upon the neocortex, MDAS and neurohormonal depots, but their clinical actions seem to correlate with their depressant influences on limbic structures, the septum, amygdala and hippocampus. Such a depression may simulate to a certain degree the tranquilization observed with animals subjected to extirpations of these structures. Another example of this inhibiting action is seen on electrical stimulation of the amygdala when the resulting evoked potentials are recorded from the hippocampus. The administration of minor tranquilizers such as chlordiazepoxide or diazepam reduces-the hippocampal responses.

As mentioned in the first part of this monograph, the amygdala and hippocampus may exert facilitatory influences upon the hypothalamus and this reduction of the sensitivity may indirectly make hypothalamic mechanisms less susceptible to stimuli, therefore diminished reactions to stressful influences, and thus ameliorating anxiety. Such a desirable clinical response also correlates with the ability of these drugs to inhibit, to a moderate degree, the alerting reaction to stimuli. In many cases anxiety and tension are directly correlated with functional disturbances in the cardiovascular system, the digestive or genito-urinary tract or the central nervous system. Such patients suffer from many complaints for which no pathological organic cause can be found. Often these complaints are long-standing and do not respond at all satisfactorily to the usual methods of treatment. On the other hand, somatic disease may be intensified and brought to light by tension and anxiety, without our being able to influence it significantly by the customary measures, until the anxiety and tension are relieved. The specific inhibitory action of these drugs on certain parts of the limbic system in doses that have no effect on other regions of the brain correlate closely with their known efficacy.

EFFICACY OF CARBAMAZEPINE IN LIMBIC EPILEPSY AND AFFECTIVE ILLNESS

In this book I have reviewed the concept of the *cholinergic limbic system* kindling and the role of anticholinergic drugs and *tricyclics* in blocking the seizure activity. Recent studies (Post; '82), reviewed the concepts of limbic system kindling and its possible relevance for the development of psychopathology in primary and secondary affective illness. The clinical and theoretical implications of these studies indicate that the anticonvulsant carbamazepine is effective in the treatment of manic-depressive illness. Carbamazepine is a *tricyclic compound* which has chemical features in common with previously known antiepileptics. This dualistic aspect may explain many of the effects of carbamazepine in clinical use. It exhibits a psychotropic action which may increase alertness and elevate the mood. Behavioral disorders associated with limbic epilepsy frequently respond quickly to carbamazepine; mental outlook improves, patients look and feel better.

Studies of patients with psychomotor epilepsy, with periodic *depressions* improved or showed complete remission of affective episodes when treated with carbamazepine; some patients with confusional paranoid episodes or with *manic* form behavior also improved. It is interesting to note that some of the patients showed psychiatric improvement in spite of inadequate seizure control. Thus, the mounting evidence, suggests that carbamazepine might have positive psychotropic effects on mood and behavioral disturbances occurring secondarily to psychomotor seizure disorders (Trimble; '85). This emerging literature was instrumental in Post's clinical trials of carbamazepine in patients without evidence of seizure disorder.

Chapter 8

MASKED DEPRESSION

The majority of patients who are treated in primary care are also suffering from anxiety symptoms, which may be expressed as somatic symptoms and mask the far more important underlying depressive illness.

In recent years, psychiatrist describe a sub-group of neurotic patients whose anxiety was not reactive, nor was subjective to analysis or treatment by means of psychoanalysis. This anxiety comprised some psychopathological characteristics with vital sadness. Neurotic symptoms, are an anxiety equivalence or an expression of an anxiety. Such a wide variety of manifestations such as anxiety in psychiatric practice poses the challenge of understanding the reason for the development of an anxiety, as Freud mentioned. If we accept that patients with masked depressions are psychosomatic patients in the classical sense, then we can understand that the theory of masked depressions incorporates psychosomatic neurotic disorders within affective disorders. This is very much in accordance with the spirit of DSM-III. Symptoms of anxiety and depression or invariably present together and are influenced by external circumstances. Together they constitute the affective spectrum.

DIAGNOSING MASKED DEPRESSION

Depressive illness has typical and atypical manifestations, the latter being the masked depression and the depressive affective equivalence. Masked depressions are defined as a depressive illness in which the somatic symptoms occupy the foreground, all in which the psychological symptoms recede into the background. This is not a complete definition because it refers only to the somatic masks. There are also psychological masks in which patients present with symptoms of other psychiatric disorders. Occasionally depressive symptoms are lacking completely; these are known as depressive equivalence. This is a concept still under investigation and should be used with caution.

Masked depressions have important diagnostic significance for psychiatrists and other physicians because most patients with masked depression consult physicians in the first incidence. Patients who have affective disorders that consult psychiatrists usually present with psychopathological symptoms, behavioral disturbances, suicidal tendencies, and a high level of hypochondriacal traits. Whereas patients visiting other physicians show more physical symptoms of depression.

Although masked depressions have been recognized for many years and have been given different names, there have been thoroughly investigated only in the last fifteen years or so, due in part to the use of pharmacotherapy. Depressive illness may have somatic and psychological masks. These psychological masks are depressive and anxious; they sometimes have the vegetative correlates of depression and anxiety, although symptoms may be modified by the individuals experience of anxious or depressive illness.

RECURRENT BRIEF DEPRESSION

The modern investigations in the normal population and in general practice missed short-lived depressive episode because their interviews and populational and diagnostics are based on the assumption of a minimal duration of a depressive episode of two weeks, as specified in the DSM-III-R. However, recent community and general practice studies whose interviews are structured to list a wide range of information on psychological symptoms, again identified brief depressive episodes of clinical relevance which appear to reoccur at irregular intervals, thus giving rise to the concept of a recurrent brief depression.

Recurrent brief depression is a new diagnostic category of depressive syndromes. The operational criteria require the presence of a depressed mood or loss of interest, with at least five of nine depressive symptoms (analogous to the DSM-III-R criteria for major depression; yet in contrast to major depression, these symptoms last less than two weeks, but need to reoccur at least 12 times over one year, i.e., approximately monthly, and lead to work impairment). In 90% of cases, the depressive episodes last one to three days, and in half of the cases, they reoccur every two weeks. However, the time intervals between the phases are irregular. Sixteen percent of the general population indicated that they had suffered at least once in their lifetime from recurrent brief depression. Taking all the studies on recurrent brief depression together, the average length of depressive episodes was one to three days. The age at onset for recurrent brief depression appears to be rather young; and the sex ratio for recurrent brief depression was 1.1.

Recurrent brief depression is not a distinct disorder, but it belongs in the spectrum of depressive disorders and represents a special subcategory of depression. Given its consequences a long-term course, it is warranted to draw attention to this particular form of depressive disorder.

DEPRESSIVE PERSONALITY DISORDER

Recently there has been a resurgence of interest in the concept of depressive personality disorder as a separate and distinctive personality disorder, and criteria for it have now been included in the appendix of DSM-IV. Kraepelin was the first to describe the depressive personality. Such people are persistently gloomy, joyless and anxious, with a predominately depressed, despondent, and despairing mood. They are also described as serious, burdened, guilt-ridden, self-reproaching, self-denying, and lacking in self-confidence. A basic difference between personality disorders and mood disorders is that mood disorders tend to be predominately distressful to the patient. In contrast, personality disorders tend to be characteristic of the patient's usual mode of functioning (i.e., trait-like) and often tend not to be directly distressful to the patient. The core problem of depressive personality disorder is excessive negative, pessimistic beliefs about oneself and other people. Many patients with depressive personality disorder did not have major depression.

UNRECOGNIZED AND UNDIAGNOSED DEPRESSION

There are many reasons the recognition and diagnoses of depression may be missed. One of the most common is that the clinicians may be reluctant to make the diagnosis of major depression in the face of highly disruptive life events that might make anyone demoralized, unhappy, or feel overwhelmed. In the context of such life stressors, individuals, their family, and even their physicians may substitute understanding the dysphoria for making the diagnoses and initiating treatment. The individual, deprived of appropriate treatment, may suffer needlessly and be exposed to all the morbid complications of major depression over protracted periods. Thus, for example, the co-occurrence of major depression with cancer, cardiovascular disease, neurologic illness, and other medical illnesses, is common but frequently undiagnosed in these situations. Similarly, non-medical life stressors may be associated with an increased risk for major depression. Among the best studied of these is "loss". Spousal bereavement, in fact, often is considered the most critical life stress event, and the one most likely to result in psychopathology.

Large numbers of bereaved individuals suffer from disabling and often enduring symptoms of subsyndromal symptomatic depressions. Over half of all widowed subjects had crying spells, sleep disturbances, low mood, loss of appetite, fatigue, and stroke or poor memory at sometime during the first year of bereavement. The general, somatic symptoms are likely to improve, while psychological symptoms, e.g., hopelessness persist. While people at all ages are vulnerable to losing significant others, bereavement is particularly prevalent during late-life, when friends, siblings, adult children, and particularly spouses may die. Depression may be relatively mild; however, recent investigators have found out that symptoms of depression are persistent and remain present in many widows and widowers at least through the second year of their bereavement.

Fortunately, major depression is one of the most treatable of the psychiatric disorders, with about 70% of all patients responding well to any given antidepressant medications. Thus, it is essential for clinicians to recognize, diagnose, and promptly initiate appropriate treatment of patients with major depression. Yet, all to often, major depression is not recognized, the diagnoses overlooked, and treatment is denied. Mood disorders (bipolar, schizoaffective, and depressive illness) are serious and common illnesses with a point prevalence of at least 5% in the general population over 18 years old. Mood disorders are, in many cases, chronic conditions causing as much disablement and mortality as other serious illnesses such as hypertension and diabetes.

Mood disorders are episodic and recurrent, with a depressive illness usually commencing in the third or fourth decade of life. The episodes of illness commonly lasts 6 to 18 months but their extent is variable. Depression is recurrent in over 70% of patients with multiple episodes and would merit long-term treatment in at least 60% of the cases. The life of these patients is severely disrupted: their working capacity is weakened, and the effect on their matrimonial or social life is detrimental. Thus there should be a greater awareness among psychiatrist and general practitioners, other doctors, nurses, or other health care workers. All patients and their relatives must also be educated about the nature and course of the illness. They should be told that episodes can last a period of 6 to 18 months but that no one can ascertain the end of the episodes except by the trial and error of discontinuing medication and following the patients carefully afterwards to insure there is no immediate relapse.

MASKED DEPRESSION

By masked depression is meant the existence of depressive states in which psychosomatic symptoms are so masked that it is difficult to recognize the actual psychopatholigical symptoms. This in no way constitutes a new form of depression. The term is an explanatory in nature. It is a didactic principle of bearing in mind the presence of a depression in the face of a physical complaint, particularly pain for which there are neither objective findings nor any somatically oriented treatment to which there is a response. In order to recognize the depression, it is advisable to become acquainted with the psychic, psychomotor, and psychosomatic elements of the syndrome. When they gain the upperhand, the psychosomatic symptoms dominate the entire picture presented by a masked depression.

Accurate diagnosis and differential diagnosis are important if only for the reason that masked forms of depression respond very well to antidepressant treatment, particularly when they are of an endogenous character. In the case of nonendogenous masked depression or psychosomatic disorders, combined pharmacotherapy or psychotherapy have proved of great value. Antidepressants are invariably the drug of choice. In fact, when there is evidence of depression; as opposed to benzodiazepine derivatives, they constitute no danger of habituation or other hazards among the nonendogenous forms of depression with attendant psychosomatic symptoms should be included exhaustion depression, which occurs after periods of prolonged emotional strain lasting a number of months or years.

It is important to be alert for masked depression, it is therefore essential that the right questions must be put to the patient in order to establish a diagnosis. For this purpose several questions have to be asked, for example, the patient has to be asked whether he feels oppressed dejected or whether at times he wants to cry. He should also be asked whether he gets pleasure out of things or does he have any less initiative in his work, spare time and whether he has interests in daily events, etc. This way also one can determine whether the patient feels or considers himself a failure and that he often reproaches himself and feeling guilty and having inferiority. Such patients also are if asked feeling very pessimistic at times and that they have the feeling that everything is pointless. One of the points mentioned by another patient when asked whether they have friends or contacts with relatives, they will definitely confirm that they have less contacts. In most cases, the patients have less appetite. They lose weight and have sexual difficulties. They usually feel worse in the morning and they have what is called early waking.

The inability of many psychosomatic patients to verbalize emotional problems and the tendency to over-rate somatic complaints are often the expression of a fear of being stigmatized. The division of disorders into "respectable" (organic) and "disrespectable" (mental) is not only common among patients; the doctor too should not be afraid to point out that his diagnosis involves a mental disorder. Added to this is the frequent difficulty of recognizing the true clinical picture presented by psychosomatic disorders. Unlike neuroses, whose symptoms clearly belong to the emotional sphere, psychosomatic disorders are primarily bound up with organic functions so that their connection with psychic processes or not at first apparent, either to the doctor or to the patient. The constant readiness to carry out a thorough physical examination and somatic elucidation should in no way prevent us, however, from exerting a psychotherapeutic effect on the patient from the very beginning. This is often really difficult for the general practitioner since his normal medical training has usually not prepared him for such a task. Despite all endeavors and the best of intentions, he scarcely knows how to act or what words to use. His dealings with problem patients thus cause him much uneasiness.

Moreover patients that are so intimately bound up with their symptoms for a long time are not easily convinced by initial attempts that suggests that their complaints may be connected with emotional difficulties. Far more frequently, they wish to hear that they have an organic disorder. Such resistance is particularly marked in patients with painful functional disturbances. This inner uncertainty leads them to seek out a doctor who will confirm the presence of a physical complaint and cure them of it. In the course of the frequent change of doctor they drive many excellent physicians to the point of desperation. This behavior is to a certain extent a side effect of social health schemes. Many patients today take the view that their disorders are a matter for the insurance people and their own doctors. The non-specialists usually hears only about the unpleasant physical effect not about the underlying emotions. This becomes particularly apparent when patients complain of tiredness and exhaustion. This they attribute to over work and external factors, even when they exhibit distinct neurotic and depressive traits. Patients often say they are tired, when they are in fact meaning something quite different. They may simply need a doctor or be nursing a secret fear of severe illness such as cancer. Frequently, they will want to hear the doctor confirm the relatively harmless complaint of tiredness and have a medication prescribed. Sometimes this symptom is "offered" as a cue or signal in order to get into conversation with the doctor.

The busy doctor is particularly prone to giving advice too hastily and at too early a stage in the conversation. Thus acting on the basis of incomplete or preconceived knowledge of the patient. His responsible attitude is first to listen to let the patient speak so that he can formulate his problem. That is as much for his own benefit as for the doctors. Very often the patient becomes aware of his worries and conflicts only when he has to explain the reason for his visit. From the outset the conversation must always have a therapeutic aim; the patient must be able to sense this, for he often wants to be treated from the moment he enters the consulting room. The doctor who knows how to listen not only enables his patient to elaborate on the symptoms but also allows him to give expression to his attitude to the world, his preferences, his hidden aggressions, and his secret desires. The patient must feel that he can talk without fear of being judged or condemned. He should feel that he can tend to be somewhat aggressive without erecting a barrier between himself and the doctor. For he does want to confide. He may perhaps come to know his deepest feelings for the first time when he realizes that the doctor is interested in him, and when he senses the doctor's aim to integrate the symptoms into his own life.

Everything the doctor says is important in gaining the patient's trust, regardless of whether he is discussing details of the illness itself, a possible operation, diet, or drug therapy. The way in which a drug is described to the patient is at least as important as what is actually written on the prescription.

The general practitioner can usually exert a greater psychotherapeutic effect than he realizes, but his knowledge of it is generally unsystematic. His full capacity in this field thus remains undeveloped. At the same time the general practitioner has excellent chances of getting to know the patient's psychosocial situation and apply his inference of his close contacts, his many patients, and their families. The practitioner needs to acquire the knowledge and skill of applying the necessary techniques and develop a therapeutic personality.

In masked depressions symptoms of anxiety are prominent, whether with somatic and vegetative symptoms, whereas the typical depressive symptoms are less apparent. The DSM-III has revised the concept of neurosis; the main forms of neurosis have either been included in other categories or constitute new ones. Neurotic depression is no longer an accepted category but is included as a form of affective disorder. Anxiety disorder, dissociative disorders and psychosexual disorders are now independent entities, although some evidence point to the strong relationship between anxiety and affective disorders. If we accept that patients with masked depressions are psychosomatic patients in the classical sense, then we can understand that the theory of masked depressions incorporates psychosomatic (neurotic) within affective disorders. This is very much in accordance with the spirit of the DSM-III. Symptoms of anxiety and depression are invariably present together and are influenced by external circumstances. Together they constitute the affective spectrum.

Chapter 9

DOES FREUD STAND UP TO
HARD PSYCHOANALYSIS?

For half a century or more, Freudian thinking dominated America. Now, even at rather traditional institutions, psychoanalysis, the most conservative of psychotherapies, is changing in response to the perspective medication brings. Freud's early work on the unconscious was denounced from the outset by the Vienna Medical Society. After the appearance in 1899 of *The Interpretation of Dreams* he was stigmatized as anti-religious by organized religion and a smut-peddling sorcerer by the popular press, which claimed his book taught only that innocent babies lusted after their parents.

People believed him a crazy man who saw sex in everything. Ladies blushed when you mentioned his name. However, after World War I, the world seemed more ready to accept the fact of sex—and scientists to accept the growing evidence which Freud and his followers accumulated to support psychoanalysis. By 1931, his 75th birthday, was an occasion for tributes from around the world—one of them from the Vienna Medical Society. The 20th century had by now acknowledged him as one of the greatest shapers of the **modern mind.**

However in 1940, in the U.S., the most important modifications of Freud's teachings came from Karen Horney and Harry Stack Sullivan. These neo-Freudians have attached far greater importance to interpersonal relationships and social environment. One of Horney's most interesting concepts was that of the "hidden" values and desires. She made the point that Freud over-emphasized sex, but agreed that sex was a dangerous topic for discussion in polite Viennese society at the turn of the century. However, in the U.S. of 1940, Karen Horney felt this was no longer true and Freud's overwhelming emphasis on hidden sex impulses was out of date.

She believed, that concealing any desire or feeling was a more important factor than **repressed sex.** By placing less importance on sex, she hoped to make Freudian analysis more acceptable to the general public.

It is to be recalled that Freud discovered that repressed experiences relegated to the unconscious exerted, by way of preconscious, a considerable "dynamic" effect on the whole personality. Events which were no longer part of the conscious mind exerted a marked influence from the other side of the threshold of consciousness. These discoveries led to the theory of the unconscious which, while inaccessible as such to the subject, can be rendered conscious by means of analysis. Experiences which cannot be handled in the conscious or the preconscious are repressed by defence mechanisms into the unconscious (displacement).

In the very early stages of psychoanalysis, the all-important discovery was made that dreams provided a means of reaching the unconscious. In addition to dreams and free association, the latter being fostered in a relaxed mental state such as is aimed at in psychoanalysis, symptomatic acts (slips of the tongue, mistakes in writing, lapses of memory, mislaying an object) also give important clues to unconscious processes. Alongside the discovery of resistance and defence mechanisms and the realization that the unconscious could be reached through dreams, free association and symptomatic acts, another methodolically and therapeutically important phenomenon also came into light, namely **transference.**

According to the law of vexation compulsion, the erotic trance to feel compelled to repeat infantile behavior in later stages of his life, even when it no longer serves any useful purpose. Because of this repetition compulsion, every patient receiving psychoanalytical treatment to a greater or lesser extent transfers his feelings to the analyst, displacing his memories to the most important people in his childhood (father, mother, and possibly siblings). The phenomena of transference and resistance, together with the Oedipus complex and infantile sexuality, are among the key factors in psychoanalysis. As Freud said: "The assumption of unconscious mental processes, the recognition of the theory of resistance and repression, and the appreciation of sexuality and the Oedipus complex constitute the main elements of psychoanalysis and the basic premises of its theory; no one should consider himself a psychoanalyst if he cannot sanction them".

The psychic "energy" of repressed experience and the dynamics of the 'mechanism' of symptom formation in hysterical and other neurotic syndromes still far more form a driving force in the individual than from conflict between the conscious and the unconscious. Freud called this force "libido", by which he understood the energy of the sexual drive. This drive, which serves both to preserve the species and to satisfy the pleasure principle, is particularly likely to come into conflict with prevailing moral laws. Even if it is repressed, it retains its original energy and may take the form of symptoms (conversion symptoms). It can lead to defused anxiety (**anxiety neurosis**) or become attached to inappropriate objects. At best, insufficient release of libido will result in *sublimation*, the originally sexual libido being converted into intellectual or artistic activity.

Psychoanalysis represents an attempt to examine the human personality in depth, going beyond the investigation of the content of consciousness. The three major divisions of the personality into the id, the ego and the super-ego was later adopted by many schools of psychology, although different terms were employed. The is is the realm of unconscious, of the instincts and the vital forces; it supports and influences the other two. The ego, which becomes crystallized during the rebellious phase, is responsible for conscious parts of the personality, self-awareness and voluntary behavior; the ego is the organized part of the personality whereas the id is the "unorganized". The super-ego conforms to the obligating—restrictive but guiding—rules of society and is therefore responsible for conscious and morality. Using the above terminology, the aim of analytical treatment as Freud saw it—an aim which he himself described as Utopian—was that "the ego should take over from the id", i.e. that the unconscious thought processes should as far as possible be uncovered and rendered conscious so that they could be integrated into the existing organization. Actual conflict, triggered off by "temptation and failure situations", is intensified by the residuum of unresolved childhood experiences. The consciousness may finally become dependent on infantile and repressed instinctual desires.

Conflict as an experience represents a clash between at least two incompatible tendencies which act simultaneously as motives determining experience and behavior. A disturbed relation to the mother in earlier life generates conflict in the patient between the "wish for tenderness" on the one hand and the "fear of tenderness" on the other. Patients are characterized by underlying anxiety with hysterical and/or hypochondriacal traits. The patient himself is unaware of such anxiety.

Students often have the impression that psychoanalytic theory is exclusively the work of its founder, Sigmund Freud, that since his death its significance is largely historical. This is untrue. Freud himself had changed his theories many times, and many others have made original contributions to the psychoanalytic literature. However, what is more important is to realize that psychoanalytic theories are very much alive as we near the end of the twentieth century and continue to be evolved in many directions.

Psychoanalysis and psychoanalytic psychotherapy apply the principles of psychoanalysis to understanding and modifying human behavior. The two forms of treatment are similar in that both examine psychodynamics, which studies the idea, impulses, emotions, and defence mechanisms that explain how the mind works and adapts. Psychoanalysis attempts to rely primarily on interpretation as its technical modality and concentrates on the transference (the relationship between the psychiatrist and the patient). Psychoanalytic psychotherapy also uses interpretation but concentrates less on the transference and more on **real-life** events. In addition, psychoanalytic psychotherapy emphasizes *current* interpersonal activities, whereas psychoanalysis tries to reconstruct the patient's past life. There is, however, a continuum between the two treatment modalities, so that it may be difficult to decide whether a particular method is psychoanalysis or psychoanalytic psychotherapy.

The chief requirement of psychoanalysis is the gradual integration of the previously repressed material into the total structure of the personality. It is a slow process, which requires the analyst to maintain a balance between the interpretation of unconscious material and the patient's ability to deal with increased awareness. If the work proceeds *too rapidly*, there is a danger that the patient will experience the analyses as a new *trauma*. The work of analyses initially is preparing the patient to deal with material that has been uncovered, which produces anxiety. The patient is taught to be aware of innermost thoughts and feelings and to recognize that there are natural resistance to the mind's willingness or ability to deal directly with noxious psychic material. The patient and analyst seldom follow a straight path to insight. Instead, the process of analysis is more like putting together the pieces of an immense complicated jigsaw puzzle.

Psychoanalysis takes time—between two and five years, sometimes even longer. Sessions are usually held four or five times a week for 45-50 minutes each. Some analyses are conducted with less frequency and with the sessions varying from 20-30 minutes.

The fundamental rule of psychoanalysis is *free association*. Free association refers to the patients saying everything that comes to mind without any censoring, regardless of whether they believe the thought to be unacceptable, unimportant, or embarrassing. Associations are directed by three kinds of unconscious forces, the pathogenic conflicts of the neurosis, the wish to get well, and the wish to please the analyst. The interplay among these factors become very complex. For example, the thought or inference that is unacceptable to the patient and that is a part of his or her neurosis may conflict with the patient's wish to please the analyst, who, the patient assumes, also finds the impulse unacceptable. But if the patient follows the fundamental rule, he or she will overcome that resistance. The analyst's counterpart to the patient's free association is a special way of listening called *"free-floating attention"*. The analyst allows the patient's association to stimulate his or her own associations and is thereby unable to discern as seen in the patient's free associations that he or she may reflect back to the patient then or at some later time.

In psychoanalysis, the analyst provides the patient with interpretations about psychological events that were neither previously understood by nor meaningful to the patient. Interpretations must be well timed. The analyst may have a formulation in mind, but the patient may not be prepared to deal with it directly because of a variety of factors, such as anxiety level, negative transference, and external life stress. The analyst may decide to wait until the patient can fully understand the interpretation. Popular interpretations of Freud's views have often distorted or over-simplified them. Among professionals, many psychologists and psychiatrists regard his theories with scepticism. Many psychoanalysts have departed from Freud's original doctrines, with the result that a number of schools incorporating modifications of Freudian principles have arisen during the last 40 years or so. The climate of controversy, the diversity or interpretation which have always surrounded Freudianism and its metaphorical language combine to make it a confusing subject for the layman. One major obstacle to understanding the doctrine is that it demands acceptance of some ideas regarding human behavior which are distasteful to most people. An added difficulty is that Freud's theories are not open to the clear-cut confirmation or disproof required by the normal scientific method, even though he built his theories and techniques on experiences gained in treating patients for certain psychological disorders.

Psychoanalytics theory has been criticized for not being testable, but it is rich in explanatory power and has influenced psychiatry practice profoundly. Furthermore, it is not true that all the theories of Freud and his followers are untestable. Psychoanalytic hypotheses may be difficult to test empirically, but the same thing could (and should) be said about any psychological hypotheses involving complex phenomena and worthy of being tested. The fact of the matter is that psychoanalytic theories have inspired more empirical research in the social and behavioral sciences than any other group of theories.

THE FOUNDATION OF CLASSICAL PSYCHOANALYSIS

Many doubt Freud's methods but his ideas have had a lasting influence on our lives. His name evokes awe and fear. But was the father of psychoanalysis really a genius? Opinions still differ as to the validity of psychoanalysis. Experimental psychologists, with the emphasis on scientific proof, tend to refer to the theory as aspired speculation rather than as a body of knowledge supported by solid evidence. The analysts reply that their critics misinterpret the theory and, moreover, insist on standards of proof that are too rigid for the difficult problems attacked daily by psychiatry. Like many other forms of healing, it can boast spectacular success—while critics continue to find an embarrassment of failure. Psychoanalysis emerges from their critique as an inefficient method of treating neuroses with no experimental support for its notions. They describe for it himself as quite lacking in the empirical or ethical scruples that we would hope to find in any responsible scientist, to say nothing of a major one. This new Freud is no longer the lone genius pioneer, boldly going where no man has gone before, fearlessly exposing the deep, dark murk of the unconscious. Rather the "unknown" Freud is altogether more human, a man driven by the desire to become famous, who interpreted evidence retrospectively to suit his theories and dismissed criticism with rhetorical flourishes. To them this man used his patients as pawns, expecting them to sacrifice themselves for the good of this new science. He seemed to care little if their lives were in tatters or even if they felt any better after treatment.

Nowadays psychoanalysis is under attack not just from people who criticized Freud, it is in institutional decline. In America fewer people are in analysis. Also, as will be discussed in the next chapter, all cognitive behavior therapies which somehow manage to sidestep the unconscious altogether, are on the rise. These new therapies do not depend on bringing to light *repressed traumas*. Meanwhile, the number of people taking drugs to alleviate mental disorders has increased. Ten million Americans alone are taking such medications. Out of these, about six million are taking Prozac and they are responding very well. Not only that recent drugs are not producing side effects, but also our attitude to altering mental states by the use of chemical substances has changed. It is widely accepted that certain psychoses respond favorably to drugs, which are a far cheaper form for treatment than intensive psychotherapy.

To be fair to Freud, he never claimed that the "talking cure " could work for everyone or that it could treat major psychotic disturbance. As he said: "The aim is modest: it is to turn neurotic misery into common unhappiness". A well-trained analyst will turn away a patient exhibiting, say, schizophrenic symptoms. Some documents donated by Freud's daughter, Anna, will not become available for another 50 years. Inevitably, though, as more and more of those documents come on stream, Freud becomes less god-like and more of a dedicated but "flawed human doctor". Just how flawed is open to question. The charges against him pivot on his theory of *infantile seduction*: the basis of what later he called the Oedipus complex. While, at first, he believed the stories that his mainly female patients told him of childhood sexual experiences, often with their fathers, he later decided that what he was hearing were fantasies. He simply could not accept that the Viennese middle-class were all busily involved in incestuous relationships with their children.

However, in recent years in America, there has been quite a great deal of discussion that what Freud heard in his consulting room was not fantasy but truth; that sexual abuse, particularly of girls, was rife and that Freud had effectively colluded to suppress this truth. How, in the light of current publications, the issue has become not whether these stories were true but whether there ever were such stories in the first place.

FALSE MEMORY SYNDROME

Some psychologists in America have gone back to Freud's original papers on seduction to find considerable doubts surrounding the patients' "memories" there recounted. This is crucial, Freud himself refers to his patient reproducing rather than recalling childhood events: "The principal point is that I should guess the secret and tell it to the patient straight out". Having done that, "we must not be led astray by initial denial". So, instead of the patient communicating with them to the analyst, we have the analyst foisting these experiences onto them. These psychologists believe that the patients did not report themselves sexual experiences from infancy—these were inferences made by Freud himself on the basis of a theoretical postulate.

The accusation that Freud fabricated his evidence is being used to give credibility to what has become known as False Memory Syndrome. This refers to the idea that memories of sexual abuse reported by many people in therapy are not actual memories but rather have been implanted or suggested by the therapist.

In contrast to the assault of Freud in the U.S., the European psychologists say: "What happened to Freudian psychoanalysis in America is the fault of American psychoanalysts; they throw things into a doctrine almost a religion, with its own dogma, instead of changing with the times". However, still in America, there are at least ten million people doing some kind of talking—and they are really based on Freudian principles, even though a lot of people who need these peace movements are anti-Freudian officially. However, a lot of people believe that they are standing on the shoulders of a genius.

It cannot be denied however that these days there is a biological bias. If there is indeed a biological bias these days, it is mostly reflective in psychiatric education studies published in the Spring issue of the *Academic Psychiatry* notes a "marked shift from psychodynamics mix to neurobiology" and the content of teaching programs over the past 20 years. It is not uncommon nowadays that psychiatric trainees will be talking more about drugs of course; they don't talk about the patients. In general, drugs would seem to bring quicker relief, while psychotherapy seems to catch up after about four months of treatment and it appears more effective for preventing relapses. As mentioned in the introduction to this book, some of the push for drugs undoubtedly must come from patients, who need some palpable sign that they are being helped. To a larger extent the drugs argue for themselves. Antidepressants generally, and Prozac in particular, have very palpable and efficient relief from symptoms with fewer negative consequences.

Such spectacular effects make the drugs vs. talk argument exercises in futility; drugs now are coming to be regarded as prerequisites. Drugs may simply be the wave of the future; they are already a force in the present. Freud, who trained originally as an neurologist and always longed for the approval of the scientific community, might regret that he could not have lived to see the next revolution, and perhaps greet it. The excitement over new drugs like Prozac is part of a trend that began in the late 1950's, when antidepressants first came into general use for depression. The movement paralleled a growing disenchantment with the slow, costly pace of traditional talk therapies. Within the U.S. National Institute of Mental Health, and in the profession itself, there were pressures to reach more people with quicker solutions. Critics have charged that the Psychiatric Association approves the marriage to biology because it is eager to bolster its medical identity—and thereby its standing with the health insurers.

REPRESSED-MEMORY THERAPY

Repressed-memory therapy is harming patients, disturbing families and intensifying a backlash against mental-health practitioners. Recently a lady checked herself into a California hospital as she was suffering from a prolonged bout of depression. During the five weeks of treatment there, her family and marriage counsellor repeatedly suggested that her depression stemmed from incest during her childhood. While the lady had no recollection of any abuse, the therapist kept prodding. "I was so distressed and needed help so desperately, I latched to what he was offering me", she says. "I accepted his answers". When asked for the details, she wrote page after page of what she believed were emerging *repressed memories*. She told him about running into the yard after being raped in the bathroom. She went on to recall being molested by her father when she was only a year old—as her diapers were being changed. Following what she says was the therapist's advice, the lady confronted her father with her accusations, severed her relationship with him, moved away and formed an Incest Survivals Group. However, she remained uneasy about these accusations. Signing up for a college psychology course, she examined her new found memories more carefully and concluded that they were false. Now she has begged her father's forgiveness and filed a lawsuit against the psychiatric hospital for the pain that she and her family suffered.

This is just one victim of troubling psychological phenomenon in the U.S. that is harming patients, devastating families, influencing new legislation, taking up court room time, stirring fierce controversy among experts and intensifying a backlash against all mental-health practitioners; the "recovery"—usually while in therapy—of repressed memories of childhood sexual abuse, and other bizarre incidents. No one questions that childhood sexual abuse is widespread and under-reported. The subject, rarely mentioned and then only in hushed tones until the 1980's, has become the stuff of talk shows, movies and feature articles in the U.S. Indeed, many perhaps millions of Americans, have jarring and humiliating memories of abuse, recollections that, painful as they are, have stayed with them through the years. But can memories of repeated incest and other bizarre incidents be so repressed that the victim is totally unaware of them until they emerge during the therapy or as the result of a triggering sight, smell or sound? Across the U.S. in the past several years, literally thousands of people—mostly women in their 20's, 30's and 40's—have been coming forward with accusations that they were sexually abused as children, usually by members of their own family.

Unlike the countless adults who have lived for years with painful memories of actual childhood sexual abuse, most individuals with "recovered memory" initially have no specific recollection of incest or molestation. At first, they have only a vague feeling that something may have happened. Others, simply seeking help to alleviate depression, eating disorders, marital difficulties or other common problems, are informed by unsophisticated therapists or pop-psychology books that their symptoms suggest childhood sexual abuse, all memories of which have been depressed. In the course of the therapy, many of these patients conjure up detailed recollection of sexual abuse by family members. Encouraged by their therapist to reach deeper into their recesses of their memories— often using techniques such as visualization and hypnosis—some go on to describe the events that seem to be so incredible. In many cases, the therapists conclude, and they eventually convince their patients through suggestion, that their repressed memories of childhood abuse have caused them to "dissociate". As a result, they appear to develop multiple-personality disorder, the strange and, until recently, rare condition brought to public attention; an order which is said to stem from repressed memories of early childhood trauma, including physical and sexual abuse.

The problem is that once these patients have been diagnosed with multiple personality disorder, they are convinced that they have it, and tend to exhibit what they think are the symptoms and often re-interpret their entire life history accordingly. Many psychologists who are critical of this movement said that "recovered-memory therapy will come to be recognized as the quackery of the 20th century". Psychiatrists fear that it may trigger a backlash against legitimate charges of child abuse. "As these stories are discredited, society may end up throwing the baby out with the bath water—and the hard-earned credibility of the child-abuse survival movement will go down the drain".

Chapter 10

COGNITIVE BEHAVIOR THERAPY

Psychotherapy remains the single most helpful means for the treatment of minor depression and anxiety. Medication can expedite treatment and has a great deal of influence on psychotherapy. Nowadays we are well aware how much personal medical care means to the patient—you talk a lot about it all the time. The doctor/patient relationship in the foreground of the therapeutic process has basic therapeutic significance in itself; it facilitates counselling.

It also creates good conditions for relaxation, clarification, self-discovery and maturation of the personality. For this reason alone we would not be completely unjustified in classing what radiates from the doctor's personality to the patient during physical treatment under the heading of "psychotherapy". The doctor must spend a little more time with the patient, talk to him a little more and on occasions introduce into the conversation a warmer and more personal note than a physical disorder would call for. This alone will afford the patient some relief.

By mitigating despair and emotional excitation, the doctor can often also reduce autonomic excitation and tension and improve muscle tone, respiration, blood pressure. This type of treatment centres mainly around building up a stable objective relationship and promoting a sense of security by ego-strengthening and general encouragement.

The cognitive behavior therapy approach centres on the notion that the way we think affects our emotions and behavior. This explanation of depression can be contrasted with the traditional view which regards cognitive dysfunction as a symptom of depression rather than its cause. For instance, the mood swings which are a typical feature of depression are brought on by the patient's own thoughts. These take the form of negative ideas concerning the person in relation to his or her environment which have been rehearsed over a number of years. As with many bad habits, the individual is generally unaware of what he of she is doing.

The aims of cognitive therapy are to help the patient to recognize unhelpful automatic thoughts and then replace them with more flexible and adaptive cognitive responses. Cognitive techniques used in the treatment of depressive disorders attempt to alter mal adapted thinking by using variable techniques including explanation, discussion and cautioning of assumptions. Cognitive therapy is a relatively new form of psychological treatment in which it is proposed that a style of thinking characterized by negative expectations is the basis of depressive moods. Hopelessness and helplessness are central features of depression and reflect a "cognitive triad" of a negative conception of the self, negative interpretation of ones experiences and a negative view of the future. Cognitive distortions are also present which bias the patient's view of reality and make it possible for him to believe in the ideas that are presented in intrusive thoughts.

Probably the first wholly cognitive approach to generate interest among behavioral researches was carried out at the University of Pennsylvania at Philadelphia, when Beck, Wolpe, Seligman and others were working.

The more sophisticated cognitive therapy described by Beck ('70; '76), which are similar in many respects to Ellis' ('62) Rational Emotive Therapy, was adopted much more slowly but has now become the most important of the cognitive approaches. Initially, this approach was mainly applied to depression (Beck; '67). In contrast to the traditional psychiatric view of depression, Beck proposed that the negative thinking so prominent in the disorder is not just a symptom but has a central role in the maintenance of depression. This implies that depression can be treated by helping patients to identify and modify their negative thoughts.

Beck proposed that negative thinking in depression originates in attitudes and "assumptions" which are laid down in childhood and later. In many situations these assumptions can be helpful, and guide behavior. For example, an assumption such as "to be worthwhile I must be successful" is likely to motivate considerable positive activity. However, the assumptions make the individual vulnerable to certain critical events too. In the case of the above assumption, failing an examination might be such an event; this would be interpreted as a major loss and lead to the production of "negative automatic thoughts", such as, "I am worthless", 'I am a failure as a person'.

Such thoughts would lower mood, which in turn increases the probability that further negative automatic thoughts will occur, producing a "vicious circle" which tends to maintain the depression. Once depressed, a set of "cognitive distortions" exert a general influence over the person's day-to-day functioning. These are manifest as the "cognitive triad": negative view of self, current experience, and future. Other cognitive changes may maintain this view once it is elicited; for example, patients selectively attend to events which confirm their negative view of themselves.

The reason behind this is doubtful. Depression results from lifelong habits of conscious thought. If we change these habits of thought, we will cure depression. How you think about your problems, including depression itself, will either relieve depression or aggravate it. A failure or a defeat can teach you that you are now helpless, but then the helplessness will produce only temporary symptoms of depression—unless you have a pessimistic explanatory style.

If you do, then failure and defeat can throw you into a full-blown depression. On the other hand, Seligman indicated that if your explanatory style is "optimistic", your depression will be halted.

The treatment described in this chapter presents an integration of cognitive and behavioral approaches. For this reason it is termed "COGNITIVE BEHAVIOR THERAPY". In this type of treatment the patient is helped to recognize patterns of DISTORTED THINKING and dysfunctional behavior. Systemic discussion and carefully structured behavioral assignments are being used to help patients evaluate and modify before their structured thoughts and their dysfunctional behaviors. As will be explained in this chapter "COGNITIVE BEHAVIORAL TREATMENTS" have now been developed for most disorders encountered in psychiatric practice, particularly for the treatment of depression.

The first central principal of Cognitive Behavioral Assessment is that the base way in which an individual behaves are determined by immediate situations, and the individuals interpretations of them. This therefore becomes the major focus of the assessment, with an emphasis on specific problems rather than global entities. Therapy sessions are highly structured. They start by setting an agenda, which lists items to be dealt with during the session. Patients and Therapists agree to the contents of the agenda. The main techniques of "Cognitive Behavioral Treatment" are techniques for identifying negative thoughts. Some patients find it easier to identify their negative thoughts at the start of therapy. However, others require some training before they can confidently identify their key anxiety-related thoughts.

There are several reasons why some anxious-depressed patient may find it difficult to initially identify thoughts.

— First, negative automatic thoughts may be so habitual and apparently it is possible that they fail to attract the persons attention.

— Secondly, some patients would want to spend an excessive time describing the developments of problems.

This may be because of inaccurate expectations about the interview, or because they have spent hours pondering about their problems and wish to share their thought. It may be necessary to remind such patients that the major focus of treatment is on immediate circumstances. At the interview it may also be worthwhile pointing out to the patient that a problem might have developed, for reasons which have become irrelevant and that entirely different factors may now be maintained.

However it must be emphasized that the characteristics of therapists which are believed to be important in other kinds of therapy are likely to be just as relevant in "Cognitive Behavioral Treatment". The patient needs to feel safe to disclose important and often distressing information. This will be facilitated if there is a warm and trusting atmosphere, no risk of censor, and if the therapist is emphatic and clearly committed to helping the patient overcome current difficulties and pessimism.

Seligman consistently found out that when people are depressed they are also pessimistic. This does not show that pessimism causes depression, only that depressed people tend to be pessimistic at the time they are depressed. It is not clear however whether depression causes pessimism or, for example, the chemical imbalance in the brain causes both conditions. This means that pessimism is fertile soil in which depression grows, particularly when the environment is hostile.

MILD DEPRESSION is probably nothing more than its symptoms. It is caused by conscious negative thoughts. There is no deep underlying disorder to be rooted out: not unresolved childhood conflicts, nor unconscious anger. However, major depression is different. It could be caused from chemical imbalance of the brain and that is when chemical treatment such as with Prozac or other antidepressants become very urgent, particularly if associated with Cognitive Behavioral Psychotherapy.

THE COGNITIVE MODEL OF DEPRESSION

The fact that cognitions influence mood does not imply that negative thinking causes depression. Depression may be seen as a final common pathway for a range of biological, developmental, social and psychological predisposing and precipitating variables. Depressive thinking does not cause depression; it is part of it. Cognitions may, however, have some temporal priority in the development of mood disturbance, and they can act to trigger, enhance, and maintain other symptoms. Depressing thoughts can keep depression going. In recent years two workers took the mystery out of depression. They showed us it was much simpler and more durable than it was thought to be. These were Albert Ellis and Aaron T. Beck.

Ellis successfully challenged the hallowed belief that Mental Illness is an enormously intricate, even mysterious phenomenon, curable only when deep unconscious conflicts are brought to light or a medical illness is rooted out. In the complexified world of psychology, this stripped down approach came off as revolutionary. Like Ellis, Beck found himself intensely frustrated in the 1960's because of the stranglehold the 4DN and Biomedical views had on the treatment of depression. Beck, a 4DN Psychiatrist, eventually found out that depressives think awful things about themselves and their future. May be that is all there is to depression. Maybe what looks like a symptom of depression—negative thinking—is the disease. Depression, he argued courageously, is neither bad brain chemistry nor anger turned inward. It is a disorder of conscious thought.

The Cognitive Model of Depression suggests that experience leads people to form assumptions or stigmata about themselves and the world, which are subsequently used to organize perception and to govern and evaluate behavior. The ability to predict and to make sense of ones experiences is helpful, and indeed necessary, to normal functioning. Some assumptions, however, averaged, extreme, resistance to change, and hence dysfunctional or counter productive. Dysfunctional assumptions alone do not account for the development of clinical depression. Problems arise when critical incidence occur which mess with the persons own system of beliefs. So the belief that personal worth depends entirely on success could lead to depression in the face of failure, and the belief that to be loved is essential to happiness could trigger depression following rejection.

The aim of Cognitive Therapy is to identify recurrent impulsive thoughts that increase in depressed mood. Also it counter balance negative thinking by getting the patient to examine the evidence for and against these ideas and in so doing, to become aware of and correct the logical errors that allow him to arrive at and sustain this erroneously negative ideas and beliefs. The aim is to help the patient challenge the underlying assumptions and find appropriate alternative ideas. The cause once activated, dysfunctional assumptions produce an upsurge of negative automatic thoughts. These in turn lead to symptoms of depression such as withdrawal, lack of interest, loss of interest, and anxiety, which promote cognitive symptoms such as poor concentration and indecisiveness and loss of sleep. As severe depression develops a vicious circle is formed. The Cognitive Therapist breaks into the vicious circle by teaching the patient to question negative automatic thoughts and then to challenge the assumptions in which they are based. As mentioned above the aim is also to help the patient to not only challenge the underlying assumptions but also to find appropriate alternative ideas.

NEGATIVE COGNITIVE TRIAD

Cognitive behavior therapy can be conceptualized as a type of problem/solving according to Melanie Fennell. Patients arrive with a number of problems, including depression itself. Depressive thinking prevents them from solving this. Tackling negative automatic thoughts is thus a means to an end, not an end in itself: the goal of therapy is to find solutions to the patient's problems, using negative behavioral strategies, but merely to help the patient to think more "rationally". The immediate target is symptom/relief. In the longer term, the same strategies are used to solve life/problems (such as situational or relationship difficulties) and to prevent, or at least attenuate, future episodes of depression.

Assessment of severity is important because it may reveal a need for alternative or concurrent physical treatment such as with antidepressants as would be mentioned in the following chapter. The therapist looks for evidence of what is referred to by Beck as the "Negative Cognitive Triad" which is seen by Beck as central to depression. This triad comprises distorted, negative views of the self and negative view of the future. Particular care is taken to elicit helplessness, suicidal intention and negative expectations of treatment, sustaining with this must be a priority.

It is crucial when working with depressed patients to ensure that helplessness and suicidal thoughts and intentions are elicited in the initial interview. Suicidal thoughts may not be regularly admitted and, where helplessness is present, should always be enquired after. Once suicidal intent has been admitted, seriousness should be assessed by gathering more details about whether or not plans had been made, what prevents the person from taking action, and so forth. Where extreme hopelessness and suicidal thoughts are present they must form the first point for intervention.

Therapists sometimes think that they should not mention suicide in case they put the idea in to patient's heads. In fact, it is often a relief to talk freely about it. Suicide is usually a response to thinking that one's situation is intolerable, and that nothing can be done to change it. Health instruction thus represents an attempt at problem solving. Discussion opens the way to consideration of alternative solutions or at the very least to an agreement that the option will be shelved until therapy had a chance to bite. Of course in such cases of severe depression not only "Cognitive Behavioral Therapy" but antidepressants should be administered and the patient followed very closely even if the patient has to be admitted in to Hospital.

A major advantage of psychological treatment for depression over antidepressant medication is that it can reduce the risk of relapse. "Cognitive Behavior Therapy" is particularly rich in this respect. In addition to teaching the wide range of depression management skills, described above, it decreases vulnerability to future episodes by undermining the fundamental assumptions on which depressive thinking is based. Evidence shows that interventions designed to reduce the frequency or intensity of depressing thoughts can have an immediate beneficial effect on mood. Normal reactions are created by cognitive processes that enable persons to perceive reality accurately.

In psychopathology, this ability is impaired, and errors in cognition are made. Aaron Beck used the term "schemas" to describe stable cognitive patterns through which one interprets experiences. Cognitive errors produce negative scematas that persist despite contradictory evidence. Thus, the psychogenic scematas may involve viewing experience as black or white, without shades of grey, as categorical imperatives that allow no options or as expectations that people are either all good or all bad.

As with all psychotherapies, the therapists attributes are important to successful therapy. The therapists must be able to exude warmth, understand the life experience of each patient, and be truly genuine and honest with themselves, as well as with their patients. Therapists must be able to relate descriptively and interactively with their patient. The first step is to help the patient to become aware of negative thinking and to recognize the relationship between it and depressive changes of mood. The second step is to help the patient to develop different ways of interpreting the events; for example, an individual may be encouraged to stand back from a problem in order to get a more objective view.

Patients are also given the chance to learn new skills, such as relaxation, and vocational and educational guidance may be given. Several clinical accounts demonstrate the impact of counselling in general practice, for example on the subjective feelings of patients and the doctor, and in addition the use of psychotrophic drugs and the number of consultations. Empathic doctors usually approach the patient with neither presumption nor commotion. Very few patients will pour out their hearts at the first opportunity, yet generally they are just waiting for someone to give them a signal to talk about their real problems - even those of a very intimate nature: they are eager for the sense of relief this will bring them. After such an encounter they are better able to bear the human distress expressed in their symptoms.

One may not dismiss a patient lightly by saying that he is not really ill, that there is "nothing really wrong" with them or that it is "just nerves". We must be fair to our patients; they deserve to have their complaints taken seriously without prejudice or reservation, even when no physical cause can be discovered.

In the beginning a neutral prelude to the conversation, consisting, for example, of a few impersonal questions about the patients generally or a short chat about the weather. Such a neutral start also means that the patient's first impression of the doctor is gained in a calm, informal atmosphere. The doctor must take note of both variable and avariable moods of expression on the part of the patients; this means not only listening but keeping ones eyes open too.

Behavioral techniques go hand in hand with cognitive techniques. Behavioral techniques are used to test and change mal-adaptive or inaccurate conditions. Overall purpose of such techniques is to help the patients understand the inaccuracy of their cognitive assumptions and plan new strategies and ways of dealing with issues. Depression is a vicious circle. It slows you down, mentally and physically. Everything becomes an effort, and you tire easily. You do less, and then blame yourself for doing less. You come to believe that you can do nothing, and that you will never get over your depression. Then you feel even more depressed. It becomes even more difficult to do anything. An so it goes on.

Cognitive behavioral psychotherapy is one of the most useful psychotherapeutic interventions currently available for depression (and shows promise in the treatment of other disorders). Studies have clearly demonstrated that it is very effective and in some cases of minor to moderate depression are superior or equal to medication alone. This would be explained in the next chapter about Prozac which I recommend that it is given only to moderate to severe depression and this can be done in conjunction with cognitive therapy.

Chapter 11

PROZAC: A FUTURE CHOICE

THE NEW GENERATIONS OF ANTIDEPRESSANTS

The new generations of antidepressants differ from the old generations either by being more specific than them or by acting predominately on other systems. Thus Prozac (fluoxetine) is a serotonin selective reuptake inhibitor (SSRI). Moclobemide is a reversible inhibitor of monoamine oxidases type A (RIMA). Of the new tetracyclic antidepressants, mianserin has a weak effect on norepinephrine and no effect on serotonin reuptake, but has a rather strong effect on antihistamine. This chapter will focus on SSRIs (See Stark, Fuller & Wong; '85).

THE EFFICACY OF PROZAC

Although effective pharmacologic antidepressant therapy has been available for nearly 40 years, most patients have been treated inadequately. The side effects associated with available antidepressants usually led to subtherapeutic dosing, premature discontinuation of therapy, or lack of patient compliance. The introduction in 1987 of Prozac (fluoxetine hydrochloride), the first selective serotonin uptake inhibitor (SSUI) or selective serotonin reuptake inhibitor (SSRI) available in the United States, represented a major advance in the pharmacologic management of depression. Large-scale trials showed fluoxetine to be as effective as existing agents, but because of its selectivity, the side effects of fluoxetine treatment were generally mild and transient and rarely cause premature termination of therapy.

In clinical trials approximately twice as many patients discontinue treatment because of side effects with tricyclic antidepressants (TCAs) as with fluoxetine. In contrast to older agents Prozac requires no titration and can be dosed once daily. It is also safer in overdose than TCAs. Numerous clinical trials and widespread post introduction clinical experience have demonstrated advantages of fluoxetine compared to older antidepressants. A recent study suggests that the use of fluoxetine during embryogenesis is not associated with an increased risk of a major malformation (Pastuszak et al.; '93).

SELECTIVITY OF PROZAC

Fluoxetine is highly specific for blocking serotonin uptake in the presynaptic cleft, with minimal or no affinity for blockade of uptake of other neurotransmitters. In general, the more specific an agent is as a neurotransmitter and the less it affects other receptors, the fewer associated side effects. The blockade of certain neurotransmitter receptors is primarily responsible for the adverse effects associated with older antidepressants. TCAs are far less neurotransmitter specific than SSUIs, blocking uptake of norepenephrine and to some extent serotonin and having variable affinity for neurotransmitter receptors. As a result of their effects on muscarinic, TCAs are associated with a wide range of side effects.

The most common, and often most troublesome, are anticholinergic effects resulting from blockade of muscarinic receptors, including dry mouth, blurred vision, memory impairment, constipation, urinary retention, and sinus tachycardia.

COMPLIANCE

One of the major problems in the treatment of patients with depression is that of compliance. The side effects associated with receptor blockade have discouraged patient compliance and caused premature termination of therapy with the older agents. In contrast, Prozac is the first agent to selectively block serotonin uptake with essentially no clinically relevant blockade of receptors. Compliance issues become even more important in light of the need for long-term therapy. However, if an acute treatment is hampered when a drug's side effects or dosing schedule make compliance difficult. Probably the main advantage of Prozac over the older agents is that it has several features that promote compliance.

The attitude of the doctor to antidepressant treatment is of great importance: when he is in doubt about the usefulness of medication and the patients are aware of this, non-compliance clearly increases. On the other hand in severe depression, especially with mood-congruent psychotic features, non-compliance can be a depressive symptom itself; the highest score in item 17 of the Hamilton (HAM-D) scale is given when the depressed patient denies being depressed at all. For these patients, non-compliance often results from their *lack of insight*.

Prozac's benign side effects profile is a major factor in promoting compliance. The low dropout rate was due to the more favorable side effects profile of Prozac. This is consistent with the earlier findings from clinical trials on efficiency. In which there were twice as many termination in tricyclic antidepressants patients as in Prozac patients. Moreover the once-a-day dosing schedule further facilitates patient compliance.

Breakthrough symptoms or relapse are less likely to occur with missed doses of Prozac because of the drugs extended half-life (24 to 72 hours). Here Prozac offers a further advantage, as even the compliant patient may occasionally miss a dose or two by neglecting to bring the medication on a weekend trip.

The once a day dose of Prozac (20 mg) daily is the optimum dose for most patients, and is associated with fewer and less severe side effects than higher doses. This fixed daily dose of 20 mg in depressed patients is associated with fewer and less severe side effects than higher doses. I found out in the majority of my patients (this was also found out by several investigators such as Stokes) that increasing the dose of Prozac too early in the course of therapy may be counter-productive. In my study patients who do not respond to 20 mg a day of Prozac in the first three or four weeks, some patients require higher doses to realize therapeutic benefit. In most cases increasing the dose to 40 mg after four or six weeks of incomplete response would be beneficial. However, in most cases patients will respond to the fixed low dose of Prozac. The dropout rate to adverse effects was significantly higher in patients receiving 60 mg than 20 mg.

Prozac requires no dose titration. In most cases the initial 20 mg per day starting dose is the full therapeutic dose. The dose titration required for tricyclic antidepressants has been one of the major difficulties limiting their use. However, as with all other antidepressants, several weeks or longer of treatment may be required for a full response to Prozac in which all symptoms of depression are relieved. Usually it takes about three or four weeks for marked response, but the patient might even respond earlier than this. Some patients are unaware of the subtle improvements in their depressive syndrome even after the first weeks while it can be observed by relatives or other people.

Prozac has *benign* side effect profile than the tricyclic antidepressants which exert extensive anti-cholinergic effects. In particular, dry mouth, constipation, sweating, visual disturbances, and dizziness which were reported more frequently by patients receiving tricyclics than Prozac. Also patients receiving tricyclics gained weight after about two months of treatment. Prozac has also particular advantages for the elderly patients because it does not result in cardiac toxicity or impaired cognitive function, two potential side effects of tricyclic treatment.

Unlike tricyclics, even the abrupt discontinuation of Prozac does not particularly result in unpleasant withdrawal symptoms. The extended half-life of Prozac and its metabolites, result in a gradual reduction in drug activity. Thus for most patients, there is no need to institute a series of gradual dose reductions. Prozac has built in safety of gradually diminishing plasma levels because of its extended half-life. This gradual decrease can be important in avoiding the withdrawal symptoms commonly associated with tricyclic. The possibility of withdrawal symptoms that happen with tricyclics can create a particular dilemma when a patient wishes to discontinue drug use immediately because of an intolerable side effect.

Prozac has revolutionized the treatment of depression, making management easy for the physician and tolerable for the patient. The drugs benign side effects profile and ease of dosing (no need for titration and once-a-day schedule) are the most prominent features distinguishing it from older antidepressants, and as mentioned above its extended half-life provides an additional advantage over the other antidepressants by protecting against breakthrough of symptoms or relapse when doses are missed. Prozac's safety in overdose is a particularly important feature because depressed patients are at a far greater risk of suicide than non-depressed persons. Prozac is not addictive...people do not crave for it... and there is no known withdrawal syndrome (Stokes; '93).

Intense investigation and widespread clinical studies have served to further confirm the advantages of Prozac. Prozac has become one of the most studied antidepressants ever prescribed. It is believed that more than 11,000 depressed patients have participated in clinical trials worldwide, and there have been over 3,000 published reports. Prozac is now the most common antidepressant prescribed by psychiatrists, and to date over ten million patients worldwide, including some six million in the United States, have been treated with this agent. The benefits of Prozac and widespread clinical experience support the use of this antidepressant as first-line therapy for most patients with severe depression. The severity of the depressions is reflected in the subject's average score of 22 with the Hamilton (HAM-D) Scale.

For most people, the most frightening of the symptoms of depression are thoughts of death or suicide. Having thoughts of death or suicide does not mean that the patient will act on them. However, it is important that the patient should discuss these thoughts with his doctor. They are a common symptom of depression, just as fever is a common symptom of the flu. During the early days of the introduction of Prozac, there had been a lot of media reports about it. This coverage had been encouraged by the Church of Scientology, a California-based group with a long record of opposition to the practice of psychiatry and the medications psychiatrist prescribe. A group called the Citizens' Commission on Human Rights, an arm of the Scientologists has repeatedly attacked Prozac. Now a days people do not believe these reports, and the millions of patients worldwide who are taking the medication successfully have proved that there is no basis to these allegations. It is now reassuring to the public that the scientific data and worldwide medical opinion support the view that there is no link between Prozac and thoughts of suicide. As mentioned above, suicidal thoughts or behavior are common symptoms of depression. In clinical trials, suicidal thoughts like other symptoms of depression, decreased in patients who responded to Prozac. More data repudiating a causal link between Prozac treatment and suicidal ideation came from a survey of about a thousand depressed patients treated by 27 psychiatrists during 1989. This study found no significant difference in the incidence of suicidal ideation in patients treated with Prozac and other antidepressants.

Use of Prozac rather than a tricyclic antidepressant in severely depressed patients may offer several advantages in clinical practice. Suicide is of particular concern in severely depressed patients, and Prozac has a wide margin of safety in overdose. Whereas, tricyclic antidepressant overdose is often fatal. Furthermore, preliminary evidence indicates that Prozac may be more effective than the tricyclics in the reduction of suicide drive. In addition, the more favorable side effect profile of Prozac may enhance patient compliance, and thus improve response rates over those achieved with older agents.

Moreover, the U.S. Food and Drug Administration's Psychopharmacalogical Advisory Committee met in September 1991 to review this issue and concluded that there is no credible evidence of causal link between the use of antidepressant drugs including fluoxetine and suicidal ideation or violent behavior. The committee's conclusion was based in part on a re-analysis of all the controlled trials involving the use of fluoxetine that showed no increased risk of suicide in Prozac-treated patients. Also, in patients who entered therapy with suicidal thoughts, Prozac did not cause a worsening of this thought and in fact these thought patterns tended to diminish with continued therapy.

In a recent meeting at the European "DECADE OF THE BRAIN" Research Conference in Paris, Dr. George Beaumont said that depression was often not recognized by doctors because symptoms were often inadequately reported due to the stigma still attached to mental illness; many patients had a tendency to somatize their distress (as I have discussed in Chapter VIII, Masked Depression). Depression sufferers are often not properly treated; 16% of patients stop psychotropic agents within one week, 41% within two weeks, 59% within a month. Also 15% of patients were usually given subtherapeutic doses and 26% had antidepressant medication for less than a month. Many patients drop out of therapy because of side effects. Beaumont said in Paris: "The tricyclic antidepressants were once considered a great discovery. But just as you don't drive a 1959 Buick when you have a 1994 Mercedes, you shouldn't use a tricyclic when there are better agents like SSRIs". Prozac is not toxic in an overdose. If a patient swallows a bottle, it's not likely to kill him, while an overdose of tricyclics will certainly kill him.

In the past people did not like to talk about (or even take) antidepressants because of the stigma attached to mental illness. That was a real problem, because depression is indeed very common. However, now people are willing to accept and seek treatment for depression. They're proud to say that they're on Prozac.

Chapter 12

THE DECADE OF THE BRAIN

Whether or not it will be possible to achieve dramatic benefit with this agent Prozac or others of its type is as yet unknown, but the fact that some positive responses can be obtained is very heartening. However, their use will no doubt spark further brain research that will no doubt stimulate other approaches to the central neurotransmitter system that could be more specific and more beneficial.

Only ten years ago, we knew of but a few neurotransmitters. Now, through improved techniques we have identified 40 substances and the search goes on. Over the next ten years, we expect to understand better how neurotransmitters interrelate and are balanced, one against the other to promote healthy functioning of the brain and body.

We will then be able to determine new ways of supplementing deficient neurotransmitters and decreasing or blocking the effects of neurotransmitters that exceed the brain's needs. Then we may be able to restore the proper chemical equilibrium in brain and body. Such restitution may be the answer to epilepsy, Parkinson disease, Huntington disease, Alzheimer's disease, mental retardation and schizophrenia. All these have been fully discussed in a book entitled *The Dementias: Crossroads Between Neurology & Psychiatry*, recently published by the author (Girgis; '92).

Ten years ago, we thought it impossible to replace or repair neurones damaged by trauma or disease. Today we know neurones can regrow, at least in animals, and transmit impulses again. The term "Plasticity" has now acquired a great deal of significance. Today, research and therapy programs show us that a great deal of lost brain function may be restored. Carl Cotman from the University of California wrote almost ten years ago that: "Studies on reactive synaptogenesis clearly demonstrate that the adult brain has an innate capacity to form new synapses in a highly selective manner". Reactive synaptogenesis means the reorganization of the cell in response to a stimulus.

Ten years ago, physicians could do little more than diagnose and observe the degeneration caused by neurological and communicative disorders. Today patients are being helped by earlier and more accurate diagnostic capabilities and by sophisticated drugs to reduce or halt the progression of symptoms. The implantation of neural tissue into the brain is a revolutionary concept of restoring neurological function. Scientists are now placing cells from the patient's own adrenal glands deep in that patient's brain in the area of the caudate nucleus. Some patients' symptoms seem to be reduced, at times dramatically.

The questions continue to multiply, not just about what is going on in the brains of patients who have received implants, but also what tissues should be implanted. Experiments on laboratory animals have shown that fetal brain cells work better than adrenal cells as implants which, like the adrenals, are not rejected either. There are, however, societal issues linked to using human fetal tissues that need to be addressed. The success of these experimental studies could mean widespread application of the implant technique in other neurological disorders such as Huntington's and Alzheimer's diseases. Fetal neurons containing brain chemicals associated with memory have been implanted in aged rat and the animal's memory improved dramatically. This finding suggests that implants may be useful in experimentally improving memory or slowing mental deterioration in animal models of Alzheimer's disease.

With effective therapy for Alzheimer's disease still a dream, drug trials continue, backed by PET scans and other neuro-imaging techniques. Insight from basic research probably offers the best hope for finding a treatment. Whereas the most important goal in medicine is the conquest of disease, the guiding principle in research is the abolition of ignorance. Medical science has in the past repeatedly applied the result of basic research to clinical problems to good effect. Over the year, it has been the interaction between scientists involved in basic research and those in clinical activities that most often yielded brilliant insights in diagnosis and therapy.

Scientists may be on the brink of finding in some patients, a genetic basis for Alzheimer's disease, a condition that affects 4 million Americans. The discovery of a gene in the mid-point area of chromosome 21 that produces plaques has created a new direction for research. A search for a genetic marker in these families is ongoing. A study of identical twins has shown that both do not necessarily get Alzheimer's disease, which indicates that environmental influences contribute to the disorder's development.

There are many new and exciting areas of research opportunity in the neurological sciences. In the span of two decades the stage has been set for major breakthroughs than has been expected in other fields of scientific endeavors. The foundation for future advances has been laid and the potential exists for reductions in the human toll exacted by neurological disorders. We stand on the threshold of enormous opportunities in the neurosciences, which should be fully exploited during this DECADE OF THE BRAIN .

More than three years ago a number of neuro-scientists in the United States, concerned with raising awareness of the importance of brain research, began a long campaign that culminated in an unprecedented decision by U.S. Congress to designate the next ten years as the "Decade of the Brain".

President and Mrs. Bush have both expressed their personal support for this resolution and, at a ceremony in the Rose Garden of the White House in early October 1989, the President himself issued a proclamation "calling upon all public officials and people of the U.S. to observe such a decade with appropriate programs and activities".

The International Brain Organization in its recent IBRO NEWS urged all nations to support this remarkable initiative. IBRO also urged its members to encourage their own government to support this decision of the U.S. Congress and to make the "Decade of the Brain" which started on January 1, 1990) a global initiative. The Society of Neurosciences has played an active role in helping this legislation become law.

The following statement by Dr. Murray Goldstein, Director, National Institute of Neurological Disorders and Stroke, announced the starting of the decade: "By signing the resolution declaring the 1990's the "Decade of the Brain", the President is calling on us the American public, voluntary associations, the neuroscientific research community and government at all levels to be activists in promoting research in neurosciences. Organizations like yours are vital in stimulating grass roots awareness that there is indeed hope through this research that we can provide people with relief from many deadly, painful diseases of the nervous system and their consequences. I believe we have already reached that all-important threshold where promises of success can be turned into real therapeutic progress and strategies for prevention. Now we must take advantage of this unique opportunity so that we can realize the clinical payoffs that mean freedom from the menace of neurological disorders".

The National Foundation for Brain Research in its report dated November 1989, indicated that: More than 50 million Americans are affected each year by disorders and disabilities that involve the brain, including stroke, addictive disorders, environmental neurotoxins and trauma. It is estimated that treatment, rehabilitation and related costs of disorders and disabilities that affect the brain represent a total economic burden of $305 billion annually. In recognition of the decade, the Board of Directors of the National Foundation for Research in Neurological and Communicative Disorders voted to change the name of the Foundation to the "National Foundation of Brain Research".

SUMMARY AND CONCLUSIONS

Almost any phenomenon—bereavement, loss of job, difficulties involving a spouse or partner can trigger off sensations of tension and anxiety. In a society where, increasingly, people are unwilling to make use of their own resources and will not tolerate disagreeable mood changes for long, the doctor is expected to provide chemical remedies.

General practitioners know they are in the front line of support for hundreds of thousands of people who have relatively minor disturbances because the stress of life they are leading is proving too much for them. They feel concerned that the whole burden of coping with this stress seems to have fallen on them. People know that doctors can mend broken limbs and they therefore go to the doctor to mend their damaged lives (the broken brain).

Doctors do not have a pill for every ill, a cure for every inconvenience of life. Sometimes, treating the symptoms is all doctors can do. They can't do what is hoped for and cure the cause. Some doctors may not realize how critical their initial response is to a new patient. An abrupt or dismissive reaction can be the final straw to a person who has found it impossible to talk to anyone else about their state of mind and regards the doctor as their only lifeline. Such patients need a considerate, human response.

Many millions of people throughout the world suffer from mild degrees of tension and depression. Only a few of them will ever see a psychiatrist. Far too often we hear the expression, "you must learn to live with it". This is not good enough.

Patients who are depressed or tense are eager to treat their general practitioner as counselor, adviser and trusted confident. However, many patients say that their general practitioner doesn't listen to them, not easily approached about emotional problems as he or she would about hypertension or diabetes. Instead, he or she relies mainly on prescribing drugs for treating emotional problems.

Most doctors, however, even if they are interested in the counseling side, would say that they simply do not have the time to talk to patients at length. Stressed patients usually find their problems difficult to talk about quickly and cannot present all the facts neatly in ten minutes. Finding the cause of anxiety or depression can be a very lengthy business, particularly if the general practitioner is unskilled at it and it is disconcerting for the patient if the consultation is ended abruptly.

Even doctors who are willing to listen find that sometimes their patients are reluctant to tell them the real reason for their depression or else have submerged their feelings so deeply that they are unaware of why they feel so low. Many patients also feel uncomfortable talking about psychological emotional problems in front of a highly qualified middle-class professional, who has only five minutes or so to spare them.

The patients are often in a bad mental state and they may frequently cloak it by complaining of physical ailments. A perceptive doctor, however, will see through the respectable medical symptoms and spot the warning sign of stress building up that the patient may not be aware of. Also, some patients want to know what sort of doctor they've got: cold, tough-minded, scientific or warm, friendly, understanding. So they try him out with a neutral symptom.

Doctors' attitudes to patients depends, to a certain extent, on their own personality; whether they are the "pull yourself together" type or prefer to adopt a bedside manner. In general though, doctors caught up in the general euphoria about the happiness pill have freely prescribed tranquilizers and antidepressants (such as PROZAC).

In Chapter X (COGNITIVE BEHAVIOR THERAPY), I have discussed at length the importance of this therapy whether the patient is on medications or not. A lot of patients are unhappy with their lives or their relationships or have goals which they haven't achieved. They may hide from their problems by asking for pills, but that doesn't solve anything. Unless they talk about what is upsetting them and get advice, they'll be on pills for years.

Cognitive behavioral assessment is based on simple principles and has clearly defined aims. The first, and perhaps central principle of cognitive behavioral assessment is that the ways in which an individual behaves are determined by immediate situations and the individual's interpretation of them. This therefore becomes the major focus of the assessment, with an emphasis on specific problems rather than global entities. This will be facilitated if there is a warm and trusting atmosphere, no risk of censure and if the therapist is empathic and clearly committed to helping the patient overcome current difficulties.

Doctors will sometimes prescribe medications in order to "please" the patient. After all, in the patient's eyes, the doctor is there to give tangible help. The very name of tranquilizers (and particularly more so PROZAC) beckons patients and doctors towards dreaming of a calm, serene existence.

Doctors also find themselves in a quandary when they are faced with patients in tears and under severe stress. Many are embarrassed or disconcerted by the emotion being shown and by the patients who show no signs of getting up and going. By handing them a prescription, the doctor can regain control of the situation and acceptably keep patients at arms' length.

Cognitive behavior therapy is now firmly established as the leading psychological treatment of patients suffering from a wide range of emotional disorders and numerous controlled trials have demonstrated it's effectiveness.

Cognitive behavior therapy can be conceptualized as a type of problem-solving. Patients arrive with a number of problems, including depression itself. Depressive thinking prevents them from solving these. Tackling negative automatic thoughts is thus a means to an end not an end in itself. The goal of the therapy is to find solutions to the patient's problems, using cognitive-behavioral strategies, not merely to help the patient to think more "rationally". The immediate target is symptom relief. At this stage an antidepressant such as Prozac is appropriate.

We have still not achieved a definitive hypothesis for the neuro-chemical basis of most mental disorders. As research in psychopharmacology moves with increasing direction and sophistication in the level of neurotransmitters there is signs that we may be advancing in the right direction. It is possible that we may find the answers to the causes of affective disorders in the not too distant future.

Antidepressant drugs were introduced into clinical practice in the late 1950's. The bench-mark study for antidepressant drugs, which subsequently had considerable reverberations, was the muticentre trial of IMIPRAMINE. Investigation of and speculation about the role of biogenic amines (brain neurotransmitters) in the medication of mood and in the psychopathology of affective disorders has occupied a great deal of attention in the past decade. In the early and mid-sixties it was hypothesized that clinical depression was associated with a functional deficiency of the neurotransmitters norepinephrine or serotonin at crucial receptions sites in the brain, while mania would be associated with a function excess of these amines. Tricyclic antidepressants, such as Tryptanol, were used for a long time although the side effects somehow limited their use and efficiency.

More recently, in an attempt to manufacture antidepressants without the adverse effects of the tricyclics, many novel compounds have been introduced. In almost every case, it has been claimed that the drug is safer and better tolerated than previous ones and that it is especially suited to the elderly patient.

Although in some parts of the world the number of Prozac prescriptions is only a fraction of those written for the Tricyclic drugs the most commonly prescribed antidepressants the extraordinary hype that has surrounded Prozac in the U.S. has filtered throughout the world. It is not uncommon for patients to ask specifically for Prozac which is unprecedented for an antidepressant.

Prozac, which became available in the U.S. in 1987, is the brand name of the chemical Fluoxetine. Since its introduction in the U.S. more than six million Americans have used it; more than ten million people have used it worldwide, making it the worlds number one prescribed antidepressant. What sets Prozac from other antidepressants is that it is the first drug to come on the market without apparent side-effects. As mentioned above, a deficiency in the brain neurotransmitter, serotonin may cause depression. Prozac prevents nerve cells from taking up serotonin, leaving more in the neurotransmission system. The effects are dramatic.

However, as reported in more detail in Chapter XI (PROZAC: BETTER FUTURE) the great majority of the patients who were suffering from major depression responded dramatically to Prozac. The results were in some patients just miraculous, particularly when compared to the tricyclic results. The majority of my 150 patients were on tricyclics at one stage. They either did not respond well or had to stop taking tricyclics because of frequent side-effects.

NEUROTRANSMITTER IMBALANCE IN PSYCHIATRIC DISORDERS

Psychiatry has not always been recognized as a biological science. Its assured status today owes much to the appreciation of the role of the limbic system in behavioral science and in fact arose *pari passu* with our understanding of that system. Research in this field may be regarded as the ultimate quest of the scientist and should lead man to a richer comprehension of fellow man and the problems of society.

We have still not achieved a definitive hypothesis for the neurochemical basis of most mental disorders. As research in psychopharmacology moves with increasing direction and sophistication to the level of the neurotransmitters there are signs that we may be advancing in the right direction. It is possible that we may find the answers to the aetiology of the affective disorders in the not too distant future.

Recent investigations indicate that central cholinergic factors may play an important role in the aetiology of depression. Specifically, a given affective state may represent a balance between central cholinergic and adrenergic neurotransmitter activity in certain areas of the limbic system, depression being a disease of cholinergic dominance (Janowsky, et al.; '72; Hofstatter & Girgis; '73; Girgis; '79). Emotion, whether normal or abnormal, has a biochemical basis since all neuronal processes are dependent upon biochemical events within the neuron and at neuronal synapses. Thus the abnormal brain function in mental disorders can be assumed to be mediated in some manner by changes in local biochemical phenomena.

PSYCHOBIOLOGY OF AFFECTIVE DISORDERS

The central anticholinergic action of tricyclic antidepressants has been sorely neglected, although it may play an important role in re-establishing the disturbed neurotransmitter balance in depressive illness. So far, the prime emphasis has been placed on the effect of these agents on the monoaminergic system in depression; the resulting prevalence of the cholinergic system and disequilibrium between stimulating and inhibiting neurotransmitters has failed to gain adequate attention. The available evidence of its simultaneous central anticholinergic action has so far been mainly inferential; their peripheral anticholinergic effect seemed to indicate that an equivalent central effect be very likely. However, not many scientists linked this possibility with the therapeutic effectiveness of the tricyclics.

It has been reported (Girgis; '80; Hofstatter & Girgis; '79) that brain acetylcholinesterase (AChE) enzyme inhibition potentiates the effects of endogenous acetylcholine (ACh) and leads to depression. On the other hand, the successful use of imipramine as an anticholinergic drug was reported in Parkinsonism. Imipramine also blocks the increase in central cholinergic activity occurring with reserpine administration (Sulser, et al.; '64). If the clinical efficiency of certain tricyclic antidepressants can be related not only to monoaminergic action but also to its anticholinergic activity, such evidence would point to the link between central cholinergic mechanisms and depressive disorders.

Perhaps the most significant aspect of recent psychopharmacological research is our understanding of the site and mode of action of psychoactive drugs. Since we are concerned with the correlation between behavior and drug action it is essential and necessary that our understanding of behavior itself should be adequate. The classical conceptions of limbic involvement in emotion, learning and memory have influenced the direction of research in psychopharmacology. Scientists have looked within the limbic system for the site of action of drugs that affect disorders of emotion. Because every drug affects to a greater or lesser degree all bodily and brain components it would be surprising if the psychoactive agents did not have many actions throughout the body but in fact the brain and particularly the limbic system are exquisitively sensitive to these drugs. Although the exact functions of the limbic system are not clear it is obvious that certain regions provide complex modulating influences on behavioral patterns that are primarily integrated and controlled at other brain sites. Psychopharmacological research should search for subtle behavioral effects reflecting such modulating influences.

PSYCHOACTIVE DRUGS AND THE DYNAMIC PROPERTIES OF ACETYLCHOLINE

Only a cursory discussion of the interactions of psychoactive drugs with acetylcholine (ACh) has been presented in the literature. It has been difficult to ascribe drug-induced changes in behavior exclusively to cholinergic mechanisms. Undoubtedly this is due in part to the wide distribution of ACh throughout the CNS. Part of the complicating relationships between drug-induced alterations in the dynamics of cholinergic mechanisms and the ensuing behavior may be dose-related. A small increase in the concentration of ACh in synapse may facilitate transmission, whereas a larger increase may inhibit transmission by maintaining the postsynaptic membrane in a depolarized state.

Difficulties in assay procedures have hindered studies on the potential transmitter roles of ACh. To date, tedious and time consuming bioassays provide the only methods by which nanogram quantities of this compound can be analyzed. Newer assays utilizing gas chromatographic techniques may alleviate these problems. The lack of a histochemical method for the determination of ACh has prevented the examination of the neuronal distribution of this amine in the brain. As a substitute, the distribution of acetylcholinesterase (AChE) has been determined. The fact that a definite correlation exists between AChE activity and ACh content in the brain has been shown by many investigators (Shute & Lewis; '67; Girgis; '73).

ANTIMUSCARINIC PROPERTIES OF TRICYCLICS

Recently some psychiatrists have considered the possibility that the central atropine-like effects of tricyclics may contribute to their efficacy as antidepressants. Unlike many antidepressants, imipramine-like compounds do not inhibit monoamine oxidase but do block certain peripheral effects of ACh. If the clinical efficacy of tricyclics can be shown to be related to a central antagonism of ACh, such evidence would also point to the link between cholinergic mechanisms and depressive disorders. In the following experimental report, the author describes this possible link.

The clinical efficacy of these drugs is believed to relate to an impairment in the uptake of norepinephrine (NE) by presynaptic nerve terminals and thereby an increase in the concentration of this amine at the postsynaptic receptor sites. This effort to develop a unifying theory for the biochemical mechanism of action of the tricyclic antidepressants is put in question by reports that some clinically active compounds do not block NE uptake.

A rational explanation for the mode of action of all psychotropic drugs cannot be offered through one unifying theory, but one that best fits the purpose of bringing together the actions of many of these drugs involves their interactions with the dynamics of central catecholamines. Nevertheless, ignorance about the identity and dynamics of other possible neurotransmitters limited reasonable alternative theories. Recent findings, however, concerning the activities of the *cholinergic limbic system* (Girgis; '80; Shute; '75) may pave the way for a new working hypothesis. Janowsky et al. ('72) demonstrated physostigmine-induced depressive mood in some of their patients and point to the possible role of ACh in the genesis of affective disorders.

Reserpine causes effects which parallel those of the cholinomimetic agents and one of its side-effects is depression. Imipramine blocks the increase in central cholinergic activity occurring with reserpine administration and antagonizes physostigmine-induced suppression of operant behavior in pigeons. In man, imipramine also has prominent central and peripheral anticholinergic effect similar to that of atropine. Although the anticholinergic components in imipramine's spectrum of activity is not as potent as that of atropine for antagonizing ACh yet this should not be interpreted as insignificant, since, with higher doses used clinically there are atropine-like side effects.

EXPERIMENTAL FINDINGS

The available evidence of the central anticholinergic action of tricyclics has so far been mainly inferential; their peripheral anti-cholinergic effect seemed to indicate that an equivalent central effect may be very likely. We have recently studied the interaction between tricyclic antidepressants (suggested to have central anticholinergic activity) and physostigmine (which enhances central cholinergic activity) in rabbits and cats. "Chemitrodes" were stereotaxically implanted in different limbic structures; physostigmine was then injected intracerebrally by means of a microsyringe (for more details see Girgis; '81; '92).

The abnormal spike activity which then appeared in the EEG records were partially blocked by imipramine. However, amitriptyline was more effective, although like imipramine it has a short-acting effect. Repeated i.m. injections of these tricyclics were needed to produce this depression on the EEG spike discharges. The results of these experiments proved not only some considerable central anticholinergic action of the tricyclics, but also a considerable dealy of onset, comparable to their therapeutic lag in clinical practice. The intensity of their anticholinergic action seemed to increase over time and appeared to replicate the time consuming cumulative tricyclics during their therapeutic lag.

The most remarkable result came from a comparison with the well known anticholinergic sedative, scopolamine, that was administered intramuscularly. Four hours after the injection, the high amplitude spike activity began to subside and within ten hours the EEG became reappeared and were maximal by the eighth day but could be completely suppressed by another injection of scopolamine. This injection was repeated four times and after two months the EEG gradually assumed a normal appearance. In another series, the combination of any occasional scopolamine injection (200 ug/kg) with a routine of regularly administered tricyclics maintained a normal, calm electroencephalogram for the subsequent period of the duration of the experiment.

The combination of scopolamine and tricyclics seems to have the advantage of a prompter effect on the normalization of physostigmine-induced EEG arousal reaction and a prolonged maintenance of a near normal electrophysiological state of function, extended beyond the normalizing effect of tricyclics alone. The anticholinergic action of scopolamine is reported to exceed those of atropine more than ten times, and its specific central action has also been emphasized. Vaillant ('80) indicated that amitriptyline is ten times more potent as antimuscarinic than imipramine. Earlier the same author showed that amitriptyline is more potent than imipramine in restoring physostigmine-suppressed behavior. Unlike amitriptyline neither chlorpromazine nor methamphetamine was effective in restoring behavior suppressed by physostigmine.

Clinical evidence suggests that amitriptyline is better in agitated depressions than imipramine and also suggests that the former drug exerts more sedative effects. In man, the "sedative" dose of a wide variety of drugs with antimuscarinic properties parallels the dose that reverses physostigmine suppression parallels the dose that reverses physostigmine suppression of behavior (i.e. the dose that exerts significant central anticholinergic effects) in pigeons pretreated with methylatropine (Vaillant; '78). In other words, the sedative effects of the drugs may depend on their central antagonism of acetylcholine.

DEPRESSION, PARKINSON'S DISEASE AND ECT

The use of atropine and scopolamine in cranio-cerebral injuries was prompted by laboratory results that indicated a high content of ACh in the cerebrospinal fluid (CSF) during cerebral trauma or after electroconvulsive (ECT) therapy. (Bornstein; '46; Ward; '50; Ulett & Johnson; '57) reported that the high-voltage slow activity observed in the process of ECT was blocked by atropine and scopolamine. Reduction of the ACh store in the brain appears to have a beneficial effect in the treatment of depressed patients and is accomplished effectively by ECT. Clearing of excessive ACh into the CSF, where it can easily be determined has been described and considered a characteristic corollary of improvement of condition of emotional depression treated with ECT.

More recently (Asnis; '77) showed that ECT has a beneficial effect on depression as well as Parkinsonian signs. There is some evidence of the similarity in the biochemical basis of Parkinson's disease and depression. There is a high incidence of depression associated with the early stages of Parkinsonism, even when the accompanying physical disability is in a mild form. The incidence of depression is higher in Parkinson's disease than in many other disabilities, including a variety of medical, gynecological, surgical conditions and spinal cord injuries.

These findings suggest that the depression associated with Parkinson's disease may be not only reactive to the illness but in some manner related to it. Another approach to the association of Parkinsonism and depression is the response to ECT. A recent subjective report (Lebensohn & Jenkins; '75) described the effects of ECT on two depressed patients with Parkinson's disease. It was the impressions of the authors that there was improvement not only in the depression, but also in Parkinsonian signs. Furthermore, Asnis' more recent case report indicates that the beneficial effect of ECT on Parkinsonian signs occurred prior to improvement in the patient's depression. The Parkinsonism did not change concurrently or secondarily to changes in mood. The extrapyramidal signs all showed considerable improvement by the third ECT, whereas depression did not improve until the fifth ECT, was administered.

These findings suggest that ECT may have a specific beneficial effect on Parkinsonian and depression which are not clear. Further understanding, however, may be gained from a consideration of the treatment of Parkinsonism with another form of antidepressant therapy. Tricyclic antidepressants were used successfully in the treatment of Parkinsonism with another form of antidepressant therapy. Tricyclic antidepressants were used successfully in the treatment of Parkinsonism in the 1950's. Many researchers thought that neurological changes were secondary to mood changes, while others believed that improvement in the Parkinsonian signs was the result of a specific effect of the drug. Strang reviewed this issue in regard to tricyclics and found that most patients who showed improvement in Parkinsonian signs also showed improvement in their depression. Strang believed that these observations suggested that the drug and both a specific antidepressant and a specific anti-Parkinsonian effect.

CRITIQUE OF A SINGLE NEUROTRANSMITTER THEORY

Investigation of, and speculation about, the role of the *biogenic amines* in the mediation of mood and in the pathogenesis of the affective disorders has occupied a great deal of attention in the past decade. In the early and midsixties it was hypothesized that clinical depression was associated with a functional deficiency of norepinephrine or serotonin at crucial reception sites in the brain, whereas mania would be associated with a function excess of these amines.

The strategy of amine depletion has in itself not produced any convincing evidence supporting the hypothesis that depletion of norepinephrine or serotonin is central to the development of clinical depression. One would have to consider the possible importance of other systems which may interact with changes in monamine function. It is perhaps appropriate to describe the neurotransmitter mechanisms underlying the aetiology and treatment of Parkinsonism.

Although Hornykiewiez's ('63) observation that brain dopamine is depleted in Parkinsonism led to the successful treatment of this disease with levodopa (Cotzias, et al.; '67) the mechanism of action of L-dopa in Parkinson's disease is still not entirely certain. It is apparent that cholinergic as well as dopaminergic neurons are important in the physiological regulation of extrapyramidal function. Hyperactivity of the cholinergic neurons system has been postulated in this disease.

The excessive salivation, diaphoresis, and seborrhoeic dermatitis probably reflects this parasympathetic hyperactivity. Furthermore, the stimulation of central cholinergic neurons by the cholinesterase inhibitor physostigmine consistently aggravates the signs and symptoms of untreated Parkinson's disease. These adverse effects of pilysostigmine are reversed by the anticholinergic drugs used in the treatment of this disease and by levodopa which also improves the diaphoresis and seborrhoeic dermatitis.

In Parkinson's disease, it is believed, degeneration of the dopaminergic nigrostriatal pathway may result in a shift of the balance between inhibitory dopaminergic neurons and excitatory cholinergic neurons, producing a relative cholinergic hyperactivity which can be restored toward normal by levodopa. Interpolating this to depressive illness, it would seem reasonable to hypothesize that central *cholinergic* mechanisms also seem to play an important role in the pathophysiology of depression. Cholinesterase inhibitor insecticides and nerve gases are known to produce depression. Janowsky, et al. ('72) demonstrated physostigmine-induced depressive mood in some of their patients. These authors point to the possible role of ACh in the genesis of affective disorders. However, a rigorous extrapolation from pharmacological studies to pathophysiology clearly cannot be made.

It is not quite clear why the limbic structures are so rich in AChE enzyme. We believe, however, that AChE has a protective function, preventing the development of bizarre sensitivity in susceptible cells. The prevalence of available AChE may ensure that the sensitivity be acetylcholine is maintained within a limited safe range. As a working hypothesis derived from the results of the work mentioned above, we postulated that cerebral mechanisms underlying some emotional disturbances may be related to cholinergic hyperreactivity or hypersensitivity, of neurons of certain areas of the limbic system such as the septum, amygdala, hypothalamus or basal ganglia. Our recent findings raise the practical possibility that pharmacological manipulation of the cholinergic limbic system could be used in the treatment of depressive disorders.

Classical potent anticholinergic agents such as atropine are not presently recognized as effective antidepressants, but peripheral side-effects may be a limiting factor in the achievement of a *desirable central anticholinergic agent*.

It is to be emphasized that the existence of non-MAO inhibitor antidepressants make one consider that MAO inhibition may not be causally related to antidepressant action. The experimental effects that are specific for antidepressant action and the desirability of the inclusion of *potent central anticholinergic actions* (such as those produced by scopolamine), remain as primary objectives in our studies which seek to characterize and select more *effective antidepressant drugs*. The analogy to Parkinsonism and its treatment, in some cases, by L-dopa as well as by anticholinergic drugs can appropriately be mentioned here. It appears that the NE-potentiating and the cholinergic-blocking properties of imipramine-like compounds are mutually reinforcing to bring about the clinical antidepressant response.

In conclusion it may be said that the catecholamine hypothesis for the affective disorders and the cholinergic theory of depression presented here may both have their shortcomings. It is heartening, nevertheless, to note that with the rapid expansion of research in the neurosciences we are acquiring sufficiently detailed information about limbic brain function to develop increasingly sophisticated and meaningful theories concerning the aetiology of some major psychiatric disorders. Our experimental findings support the hypothesis that tricyclics, in addition to their well known monoaminergic action, also have a marked balancing and synergistic central anticholinergic compound of activity which may play an important role in the therapy of endogenous depression.

AFFECTIVE DISORDERS AND THE DEMENTIAS: PSEUDODEMENTIA

As indicated earlier, old age has many dangers. One is that of being regarded as demented and particular of suffering from Alzheimer's disease. "In an appreciable number of patients although they prove to have dementia full investigation discloses that the condition is treatable. Others prove not to be demented at all and retrospectively these are referred to as having pseudodementia" (Kiloh; '81). The overlap between dementia and depression can present a difficult diagnostic challenge.

Two types of overlap occur: In the first type, depressed mood with or without other features of depressive illness is part of an otherwise clearly *organic dementia*. In the second type, reversible cognitive deficits of the kind classically associated with organicity (such as memory disturbance or confusion) are found in functional depressive illness. This latter syndrome, known as depressive pseudodementia, is particularly perilous. It can lead to misdiagnosis of irreversible dementia, which may lead to the withholding of treatment, institutionalization and a downward spiral of social withdrawal, isolation and increasing depression.

The clinical picture of dementia may be mimicked by neurotic disorders notably hysteria, depression and obsessional states, by mania, schizophrenia and delirium, but most commonly by *endogenous depression*. The differential diagnosis is not made easier by the fact that a dementing process may present with depression as can many varieties of localized cerebral disease. Old people are particularly vulnerable to the misdiagnosis of dementia, for the doctor's level of expectation is high and his critical faculties may be blunted if he places undue emphasis on age as an aetiological factor.

ENDOGENOUS DEPRESSION IN THE ELDERLY

Although there is no method for reversing the basic processes of dementia in many patients, the health care system can do much to improve the quality of life for both the patient and the family. However, a significant proportion perhaps a fifth of patients with apparent dementia do have *reversible* illness. Recognition and treatment of these patients, using a systematic diagnostic process, can be one of the most gratifying experience in geriatric medicine. The systematic process begins with an awareness of the possible causes of reversible dementia. Many clinical disorders in the elderly can cause a dementia as the principal clinical manifestation and be far from obvious.

Of the patients with reversible causes, about one third were found to have pseudodementia, a form of depression. The overlap between dementia and depression can present a difficult diagnostic challenge. A diagnosis of dementia is often made by doctors who expect all old people to be demented. Pseudodementia, by definition, is not a syndrome in its own right and because dementia is common in the old, many doctors simply take its presence for granted. The impairment of memory and poor orientation that inspire the suspician of dementia may stem from the poor concentration, loss of interest and retardation due to depression.

If the loss of interest extends to personal habits with neglect of the person this only strengthens the illusion of determination and if, as is not uncommon, the patient stresses somatic symptoms and fails to mention or even denies depression, the correct diagnosis may not even be considered. The memory loss which occurs in depressed elderly patients is so significant that it poses one of the major problems in differential diagnosis for geriatric psychopathology. Indeed, the term pseudodementia has the restricted meaning of depression masquerading as dementia. Moreover, complaints of memory loss are usually not rare among geriatric depressed patients.

Endogenous depression is very difficult to differentiate from dementia. It can present in many different ways and can be influenced by concomitant diseases. Kiloh ('81) emphasizes that we should "always suspect depression, even if it is present with dementia, and treat it." It can often be recognized by abrupt onset of short duration before the time of first referral.

Dementia, on the other hand, has a slow onset and is usually not referred until 12-18 months after the first symptoms are noticed. "Depressive pseudodementia is most dangerous and has a very high mortality, even when suicide figures are discounted" (Kiloh; '81). Mortality is often the result of lack of treatment through failure to recognize the existence of depression. Kiloh indicates that ECT is usually more effective in treating depression than drugs and should always be used if there is any doubt.

THE CHOLINERGIC SYSTEM IN ALZHEIMER'S DISEASE

In the midst of the gloomy prospects concerning the social problems of the dementias, recent research on neurotransmitter systems has provided new and hopefully brighter horizons. In particular, the discovery, just six years ago, of major losses of Cholinergic activities in the brains of affected cases. A reduced concentration of choline acetyltransferase (CAT) is the biochemical abnormality confirmed most often in brain tissue affected by Alzheimer's disease. This enzyme catalyzes the acetylation of Choline to acetylcholine. The degree of this reduction, which may reach 95% of control values, has been positively correlated with the density of neurofibrillary tangles (Davies & Maloney; '76) and senile plaques, and the degree of dementia (Perry, et al.; '78). This finding has led to the hypothesis that Cholinergic cells are specifically affected in Alzheimer-associated dementia.

Several indirect lines of evidence support this hypothesis: anticholinergic drugs (scopolamine) can produce a transient memory deficit similar to that found in Alzheimer-associated dementia, and this deficit can be acutely reversed by Choline, or by physostigmine (Bartus; '78). Also administration of Choline or its dietary source, lecithin, raises concentrations of acetylcholine in the brain and enhances some aspects of memory in experimental animals or normal humans. However, in early clinical trials none of these interventions produced consistent improvement in demented patients. A possible explanation for these early disappointing results may be associated with impaired Cholinergic receptor function. Reisine et al. ('78) reported decreased numbers of ACh receptors in the hippocampus but not in other areas of Alzheimer-affected brain. In a series of related experiments Lippa et al. ('80), studying aged, memory-impaired rats, found decreased receptor responsiveness to iontophoretically applied acetylcholine, but not to glutamate. The degree of reduced responsiveness exceeded (50% compared with 20%) the degree of reduction in number of ACh receptor sites found in the same tissue.

Notable among research group working in this fundamental areas of research, who have recently turned their attention to the problem of Alzheimer's disease is that of Joseph Coyle and his co-workers at Johns Hopkins University. Previous animal experiments of theirs and others, on a Cholinergic nucleus which supplies axons to the neocortex, have demonstrated a decreased cortical Cholinergic enzyme activities following lesions in this area. This *nucleus (of Meynert)* is composed of a group of large neurons in the basal forebrain lying in an area ventral to the pallidum. Clinically, it was reported that over 75% of cells are lost in dementia.

ALZHEIMER'S DISEASE: THE CHOLINERGIC SYSTEM

New Drug Gives Hope

Basal Forebrain Cholinergic System: The cholinergic system has been show to play an important role in the processing learning, memory and cognition. The most consistent and persuasive evidence of a significant neurotransmitter deficit in Alzheimer Disease is in studies of the cholinergic system. The distribution of cholinergic neurons within the ventral forebrain has been studied extensively (Girgis; '73; '78; '80; '80a; '81). The most consistent deficiency in brains of patients with Alzheimer's disease is a reduction of presynaptic cholinergic markers in the neocortex and hippocampus, including activity of the acetylcholine synthesizing enzyme, cholineacetyltransferase (ChAT).

The significance of a ChAT deficiency is based on the observation that ChAT is localized in cholinergic neurons, and as such a marker of cholinergic neurons. It appears that the most substantial reduction of this enzyme activity occurs in frontal and temporal cortex as well as the amygdala and hippocampus. These limbic areas are of course linked to learning and memory. Recent work has shown substantial reductions in cholinergic neurons in the nucleus balsas of Meynert in the brains of patients who died from Alzheimer's Disease. These large cells project topographically to the entire neocortex. As will be shown below, drugs that impair function of the cerebral cholinergic system produce performance deficits, and drugs that potentiate central cholinergic function enhance recent memory.

In Alzheimer's Disease, the presence of apparently normal sensory, motor, and motivational behavior indicates that the widespread impairments in behavioral tasks that assess learning and memory are not due to fundamental problems in nonassociative processes such as perception, motivation, and motor coordination. Rather, these impairments must result from a fundamental disorder of cognitive mechanisms normally involved in learning and memory. These impairments are similar to those seen following damage to the temporal lobe structures that are often implicated in learning and memory. The clinical symptoms and history of a gradual worsening of the condition are used to distinguish Alzheimer's Disease from other dementing conditions. However, conclusive diagnosis can only be made by histological studies which include degeneration of cholinergic nerve cells.

The Cholinergic Hypothesis of Alzheimer's Disease: The first clear relationship to be established between age related loss of memory and related cognitive functions and a dysfunction of neurotransmission involved the cholinergic system. The logic and empirical support for this idea has become known as the cholinergic hypothesis, which asserts that significant functional disturbances in cholinergic activity occur in the brains of aged and especially demented subjects. These disturbances play an important role in the memory and related cognitive problems; and the enhancement or restoration of cholinergic function may significantly reduce the severity of cognitive loss.

The cholinergic hypothesis might be criticized as being a bit simplistic and as failing to produce effective treatment for the memory disturbances of dementia. However, the evidence that implicates an important role of this neurotransmitter seems to be quite compelling It is clear that more neurotransmitter systems must be investigated to find out whether or not Alzheimer's disease really is a condition in which there is a specific degeneration of certain cholinergic neurons. For now, this seems to be the best working hypothesis available.

Cholinergic & Anti-cholinergic Drugs and Memory: In contrast with other neurotransmitters, the role of acetylcholine in learning and memory has been bolstered by the result of clinical pharmacological studies. Pharmacologically induced alterations in central cholinergic activity produce profound changes in learning and memory. The effects of scopolamine, an anti-muscarinic agent, on learning and memory have been studied by a number of investigators Scopolamine in low does showed a deficit in the ability to learn new information and selectively reduced the encoding of new information into long term memory. Atropine had a similar effect on memory. Also scopolamine produced memory deficits in normal young subjects and these deficits were reversed by physostigmine (see below). Thus, blocking central cholinergic transmission produces one of the main symptoms of Alzheimer's Disease: difficulty learning new information.

THERAPEUTIC CHOLINERGIC STRATEGIES

Treatment with PHYSOSTIGMINE : Pharmacologic mimicking by anticholinergics of the core symptoms of Alzheimer's Disease and enhancement of memory and cognition by cholinomimetic agents support a cholinergic deficit theory in Alzheimer's Disease. These findings strongly supported therapeutic cholinergic strategies. Inhibiting breakdown of synaptic acetylcholine is the basic approach to augmentation of central cholinergic activity. Physostigmine is a reversible acetylcholinesterase inhibitor. This strategy is dependent upon intact presynaptic neurons. However, the acetylcholinesterase inhibitor does not require the presynaptic neuron to augment acetylcholine synthesis.

Acetylcholinesterase inhibition has the additional benefit of increasing activity of both nicotinic and muscarinic cholinergic receptors. Since there is some evidence implicating nicotinic activity in cognition. There is an obvious advantage to a non-specific agent. Characteristic pharmalogic effects of these inhibitors are primarily due to the prevention of acetylcholine hydrolysis at cholinergic sites.

Physostigmine is representative of the reversible inhibitors and has been extensively evaluated in several neuro-psychiatric disorders including Alzheimer's Disease. The effect, however may be short-lived particularly when administered alone. Given alone, it prolongs the life of intrasynaptic acetylcholine but will thereby diminish the formation by hydrolysis of free choline available for reuptake into the presynaptic neuron. Wurtman indicated that "protection against this possible side effect could be provided by co-administering a source of supplemental choline" (Maurer & Wurtman; '89). Physostigmine has a very short half-life, accordingly a long acting drug (THA) is now being used as will be explained below.

Treatment with THA (Tacrine): In the past, irreversible organophosphate inhibitors were found to be effective in animals for learning experiments. Diisopropylfluorophosphate (DFP), a noncompetitive acetylcholine esterase inhibitor, has in the past been administered to patients with neuro-psychiatric disorders. Such irreversible inhibitor has side effects, such as neuropathy, which cannot be prevented by atropine. THA (Tetra-hydro-aminoacridine) is a competitive acetylcholinesterase inhibitor with a half-life intermediate between physostigmine and DFP. It appears to be safe and with minimal cardiac or peripheral cholinergic effects. Liston et. al. (Neuroscience Abst. Oct., '89, p. 860) made a comparison study between THA and physostigmine. As expected, they found that THA achieve a higher concentration in the brain and has longer duration.

Tacrine is usually given to patients who have no history of stroke or hepatic disease and who, apart from their dementia, are reasonably healthy. Although the lethal dosage in man has not been established, estimates based on animal studies suggest that the lethal dose of THA would be about 30 mg/kg when unopposed by anticholinergic agents. An extensive review of human trials with THA supports its high therapeutic to toxic ratio and index of safety. Lecithin is usually given at the time; this will provide a precursor loading of choline and thereby make the THA more effective as mentioned above when discussing physostigmine.

THA has few side effects; the only common ones being nausea and occasional diarrhea. In some patients it has been reported to cause abnormalities of liver enzymes which reverse if the drug is ceased.

GENE THERAPY'S BRAVE NEW WORLD

Some 3,000 disorders are caused at least partly by defective genes or chromosomes. Gene therapy research is progressing in leaps and bounds, but it could have some alarming implications. Just as scientists have discovered that genes predispose humans to deadly diseases such as Huntington's, Alzheimer's disease and Cystic Fibrosis; the focus now is on the genes we inherit from our parents which can make us depressed, violent, alcoholic, obese, etc. The research is raising serious moral questions about whether people should be told their gene fortunes and, furthermore, whether science should be used to change how people look, feel and act.

Genetic engineering: the deliberate manipulation of genetic material by biochemical techniques which can breed functionally specific plants or animals, has been going on for some time now. In the U.S. 52 gene therapy studies have been approved in patients with diseases such as cancer and Cystic Fibrosis. In some studies, scientists are investigating how to make cancer cells more vulnerable to drugs and how to give people a health, functioning gene to compensate for a missing or faulty one. Three years ago, doctors at the National Institute of Health used gene therapy for the first time to correct an inherited disorder.

Dr. Ted Reich, a psychiatrist at Washington University's School of Medicine in St. Louis, Missouri, is investigating whether similar genetic tinkering can help alcoholics and people suffering depression. Similar research is being conducted for the socially crippling depression called Bipolar Affective Disorder (suffered by Winston Churchill and Abraham Lincoln). In four American cities, scientists are interviewing 1,600 members of 200 families and taking blood samples to find out if a gene or a group of genes predisposes a person to become depressed. Dr. Reich indicated that, if we find the genes, the next step will be to isolate the region of the chromosome that is defective and then see what it does and then work out how to treat it. Dr. Elliot Gershon, a psychiatrist at the National Institute of Mental Health in Washington, D.C., is convinced that if behavior is found to be linked to a gene or genes it should be viewed no differently for medical problems that affect vital organs.

Is there a gene that will make a person murder? Do the genes you inherit increase your chances of committing crimes? While there is no doubt that the environment people are raised in affects their behavior, some psychologists are studying whether people can inherit a predisposition to violence. While the genetic makeup of pedophiles and repetitive rapists has not been studied, there appears to be evidence for a genetic link between anti-social behavior and aggression. Some psychologists emphasize that we already know a major indicator for violence (referring to the Y chromosome only men inherit), which some scientists believe partly explains why men are generally more aggressive than women. It is believed that people with genetic makeup are nine times more likely to be arrested than those without it. But, of course, we can't go pointing the finger at every man just because they are more likely than women to be violent.

The genetic principles described above provide only a preliminary foundation for understanding inherited propensities to certain behaviors. It is specific brain proteins, finally, that control the cellular functions underlying behavior; if only one of these proteins is abnormal, it may cause or predispose to specific mental illness. It is necessary to deal with molecules in order to appreciate psychiatry. Samuel Barondes ('92), a psychiatrist at the University of California, San Francisco, recently said: "Supported by the huge growth of molecular, genetic, and cellular research, the biological approach to psychiatry is making tremendous strides." The recent burst of knowledge in the field of genetics, molecular biology, and neuroscience has begun to yield important insights that are applicable to psychiatry. It now seems reasonable to expect that a more powerful biology will provide the tools to solve some of psychiatry's most refractory problems.

RECENT ADVANCES IN BIOPSYCHIATRY

A Lab Test For Suicide!? - Sounds incredible, yet it is only one of the promising developments being pursued in the hot new field of biological psychiatry. What was once the purview of psychoanalysts who try to probe the mind by listening and observing, is now a frontier for neuroscientists who use blood tests and brain scans.

There has never been a laboratory test that doctors could order that would help them measure the risk of suicide more precisely. Suicide is the eighth leading cause of death in the U.S. When it comes to determining an individual's desire to commit suicide, physicians rely heavily on experience and intuition. That predicament seems likely to change in the next few years, as neuroscientists learn more about the biochemistry of the brain and behavior.

Some of the latest research—parts of which were presented at the November '94 meeting of the Society for Neuroscience in Miami—suggests that measuring the levels of certain chemicals in the brain can identify those people with a biological predisposition to suicide. According to John Mann of the Columbia University and New York State Psychiatric Institute: "more than 95% of the people who commit suicide show changes in the brain at autopsy. But the biochemical abnormality is there even in those who attempt to kill themselves, and it is most pronounced in those who make the most dangerous attempts."

Not everyone who is depressed attempts suicide; nor does low serotonin level automatically doom a person to self-destruction. According to John Mann, changes must occur in the orbital cortex (part of the limbic system of the brain). As I have mentioned in Chapter I (p. 9), 50% of all people who commit suicide visit their doctor in the month prior to their death. Doctors may someday be able to give these people a blood test that measures their body's ability to manufacture serotonin. Those whose capacity is impaired would be considered at greatest risk of hurting themselves. Finally, it can be said that the push to discover the biological markers of behavior shows no signs of abating. We stand on the threshold of enormous opportunities in the neurosciences, which should be fully exploited during this *'Decade of the Brain'*.

REFERENCES

Adamec, R., Stark-Adamec, C, Perrin, R. and Livingston, K.E. (1980). Limbic kindling and complex partial seizures: New strategies for detection of neurobehavioral change. *Limbic Epilepsy and the Dyscontrol Syndrome*, Girgis, M. & Kiloh, L.G. (Ed.), pp. 119-132. Elsevier/North Holland, Amsterdam.

Alonso-de Florida, F. and Delgado, J.M.R. (1958). Lasting behavioral and EEG changes in cats induced by prolonged stimulation of amygdala. *Am. J. Physiol.*, 193: 223-229.

American Psychiatric Association. (1994). *Diagnostic and Statistical Manual of Mental Disorders*, IV ed. Washington DC: APA.

Andreason, N.C. (1984). *The Broken Brain*, Harper and Row, New York.

Antidepressant Update. (1991). Food and Drug Administration, U.S. Department of Health Services Publication T91, Rockville, Md.

Arnold, P.S., Racine, R.J. and Wise, R.A. (1973). Effects of atropine, 6-hydroxydopamine and handling on seizure development in the rat. *Exp. Neurol.*, 40: 457-470.

Asnis, G. (1977). Parkinson's Disease, Depression and ECT: A Review and Case. *Amer. J. Psychiat.*, 134: 191-195.

Atkinson, R.L. (1990). *Introduction to Psychology*, HBJ Publishers, New York.

Baldwin, M. and Bailey, P. (1958). *Temporal Lobe Epilepsy*, Charles C. Thomas, Springfield.

Barondes, Samuel H. (1992). *Molecules and Mental Health Illness*, Scientific American Library, W.H. Freeman & Co., New York.

Bartus, R.T. (1978). Evidence for a direct cholinergic involvement in the scopolamine induced amnesia in monkeys: effects of concurrent administration of physostigmine and methylphenidate with scopolamine. *Pharmacol. Biochem. Behav.*, 9: 833-836.

Beck, A.T., Shaw, B.T.F. and Emery, G. (1979). *Cognitive Therapy of Depression*, Guildford Press, New York.

Beck, J.C. (1982). Dementia in the elderly: the silent epidemic. *Annals of Internal Medicine*, 97: 231-241.

Beckstead, R.M. (1979). *Neuroscience Letters*, 12: 56-69.

Belluzzi, J.D. (1972). Long-lasting effects of cholinergic stimulation of the amygdaloid complex in the rat. *J. Comp. and Physiol. Psych.*, 80: 269-282.

Ben-Ari, Y., Tremblay, E., Ottersen, O.P. and Meldrum, B.S. (1980). The role of epileptic activity in hippocampal and remote cerebral lesions induced by kainic acid. *Brain Res.,* 191: 79-97 .

Ben-Ari, Y., Zigmond, R.E., Shute, C.C.D. and Lewis, P.R. (1977). Regional distribution of choline acetyltransferase and acetylcholinesterase within the amygdaloid complex and stria terminalis system. *Brain Res.,* 120: 435-444.

Benson, D.F. (1982). Dementia in the elderly: the silent epidemic. *Annals of Internal Medicine,* 97: 231-241.

Bornstein, M. (1946). Presence and action of ACh in experimental brain trauma. *J. Neurophysiol.,* 9: 349-366.

Broca, P. (1878). Anatomie comparée des ci rcomvolutions cérébrales. I. Le grand lobe limbique et la scissure limbique dans la serie des mammifers. *Rev. d'Anthropol.,* 2nd series, 1: 385-498.

Burchfiel, J.L.K. (1979). Neuronal supersensitivity to acetylcholine induced by kindling in the rat hippocampus. *Sci ence,* 204: 1096-1098.

Butcher, L.L. (Ed) (1978). *Cholinergic-monoaminergic Interactions in the Brain,* Academic Press, New York.

Cannon, W.B. and Rosenblueth, A. (1949). *The Supersensitivity of Denervated Structures: a Law of Denervation,* Macmillan, New York, pp . 254.

Cannon, W.B.A. (1939). A law of denervation. *Amer. J. Med. Sci.,* 198: 737-750.

Celesia, G.G. and Jasper, H.H. (1966). Acetylcholine released from cerebral cortex in relation to state of activation neurology. 16: 1053-1064.

Celesia, G.G. and Wanamaker, W.M. (1972). Psychiatric disturbances in Parkinson's Disease. *Dis. Nerv. Syst.,* 33: 577-583.

Chan-Palay, V. (1976). Serotonin axons in the supra and subependymal plexuses and in the leptomeninges, their roles in local alteration of cerebrospinal fluid and vasomotor activity. *Brain Res.,* 102: 103-130.

Chatrian, G.E. and Chapman, W.P. (1960). Electrographic study of the amygdaloid region with implanted electrodes in patients with temporal lobe epilepsy. *Electrical Studies on the Unanaesthetized Brain.* Ramey, E.R. & O'Doherty, D.S. (Eds.), P.B. Hoeber, Harper.

Chu, N.S., Rutledge, L.T. and Selinger, O.Z. (1971). The effect of cortical undercutting and long-term electrical stimulation on synaptic acetylcholinesterase. *Brain Res.,* 29: 323-330 .

Conrad, S.W. (1962). Management of obesity, *Psychosomatic Medicine,* (Chpt. 110), J.H. Nodine and J.H. Moyer (Eds.), Lea & Febiger, Philadelphia.

Coppen, C.W. (1967). The biochemistry of affective disorders. *Brit. J. Psychiat.*, 113: 1237-1264.

Cotman, C.W. and Lynch, G.S. (1976). Reactive synaptogenesis in the adult nervous system: The effects of partial deafferentation on new synapse formation. *Neuronal Recognition*, S. Barondes (Ed.), Plenum Press, New York.

Cotzias, G.C., Van Woert, M.H. and Schiffer, L.M. (1967). Aromatic amino-acids and modification of Parkinsonism. *New Eng. J. Med.*, 276, 374-379.

Coyle, J.T., McGeer, E.G., McGeer, P. and Schwarcz, R. (1978). *Kainic Acid as a Tool in Neurobiology*, E.G. McGeer, J.W. Olney and P.L. McGee (Eds.), Raven Press, New York.

Cragg, B.G. (1967.) Are there structural alterations in synapses related to functioning. *Proc. R. Soc. B.*, 171: 319.

Curtis, D.R. and Johnston, G.A.R. (1974). Amino acid transmitters in the mammalian central nervous system. *Ergebn. Physiol.*, 69: 97-188.

Davies, P. (1979). Neurotransmitter-related enzymes in senile dementia of the Alzheimer's type. *Brain Research*, 171: 319327.

Davies, P. and Maloney, A.J.F. (1976). Selective loss of central cholinergic neurons in Alzheimer's disease (Letter). *Lancet*, 2: 1403.

Delgado, J..M.R. (1964). Free behavior and brain stimulation. *International Review of Neurobiology*, Vol. VI, 349-449, C.C. Pfeiffer and J.R. Smythies (Eds.), Academic Press, New York.

Delgado, J.M.R., Rivera, M.L. and MIR, D. (1971). Repeated stimulation of amygdala in awake monkeys. *Brain Res.*, 27: 111.

Domino, E.F. (1962). Human pharmacology of tranquilizing drugs. *Clin. Pharmacol. Ther.*, 3: 599-664.

Eccles, J.C., Fatt, P. and Koketsu, K. (1954). Cholinergic and inhibitory synapses in a pathway from motor-axon collaterals to motorneurones. *J. Physiol.*, 126: 524-562.

Eccles, J.C. (1966). Conscious experience & memory. *Brain and Conscious Experience*, J.C. Eccles (Ed.), Springer-Verlag, New York.

Echlin, F.A. and Battista, A. (1963). Epileptiform seizures for chronic isolated cortex. *Arch. Neurol.*, 9: 154-170.

Egger, M.D. and Flynn, J.P. (1963). Effect of electrical stimulation of the amygdala in hypothalamically elicited attack behaviour in cats. *J. Neurophysiol.*, 26: 705-720.

Ellis, A. (1962). *Reason and Emotion in Psychology*. Lyle Stuart, New York.

Engel, J. and Sharpless, N.S. (1977). Long-lasting depletion of dopamine in the rat amygdala induced by kindling stimulation. *Brain Res.*, 136: 381-386.

Ervin, F.R., Epstein, A.W. and King, H.E. (1955). Behavior of epileptic and non-epileptic patients with temporal spikes. *Arch. Neurol. Psychiat.*, 74: 488-497.

Ervin, Mark, V.H. and Stevens, J.R. (1968). Behavioral and effective responses to brain stimulation in man. *Am. Psychopathol. Assoc. Trans.*

Falconer, M.A., Hill, D., Meyer, A. and Wilson, J.L. (1958). Clinical radiological and EER correlations with pathological changes in temporal lobe epilepsy and their significance in surgical treatment. *Temporal Lobe Epilepsy*, 396-.

Fennell, M.J.V. (1989). *Depression: In-cognitive Behavior Therapy*, Hawton, K. (Ed.), Oxford Med. Pub.

Freud, Sigmund. (1933). New introductory lectures in psychoanalysis. *The Standard Edition of Complete Psychological Works of Sigmund Freud*, Vol. 22, James Strachey (Ed.), Hogarth Press, London, 1966.

Gastaut. (1953). So-called "psychomotor" and "temporal" epilepsy, *Epilepsia III*, 2: 59-96, Academic Press, New York.

Girgis, M. (1967). Distribution of cholinesterase in the basal rhinencephalic structures of the coypu (Myocaster Coypus). *J. Comp. Neurol.*, 129: 85-96.

Girgis, M. (1971a) The role of the thalamus in the regulation of aggressive behavior. *Int. J. Neurol.*, 8: 327-351.

Girgis, M. (1971b). The orbital surface of the frontal lobe of the brain and mental disorders. *Acta Psychiat.*, Scand., Suppl. 222.

Girgis, M. (1978). Neostigmine-activated epileptiform discharge in the amygdala: Electrographic-behavioral correlations. *Epilepsia*, 19: 521-530.

Girgis, M. (1980). Participation of muscarinic cholinergic receptors may be an important requirement of the kindling process. *Exp. Neurol.*, 70: 458-461.

Girgis, M. (1981a). Neuronal hypersensitivity to acetylcholinesterase inhibitors induced by a kindling stimulus. *Brain Res.*, 207: 1-8.

Girgis, M. (1981b). Electrical versus cholinergic kindling. *Electroenceph. and Clin. Neurophysiol.*, 51: 417-425.

Girgis, M. (1981c). *Neural Substrates of Limbic Epilepsy*, Warren H. Green Inc., St. Louis.

Girgis, M. (1982). Ammon's Horn necrosis as a result of amygdaloid seizure discharge in temporal lobe epilepsy. *Advances in Epileptology*, XIII, H. Akimoto, H. Kazamatsuri, M. Seino and A. Ward (Eds.), Raven Press, N.Y.

Girgis, M. (1985a). The role of neurotoxins in the brain damage associated with limbic epilepsy. *J. of Neurology*, Vol. 232: 17, 30, 18.

Girgis, M. (1985b). Neurochemical basis of limbic epilepsy. *The Psychopharmacology of Epilepsy*, Trimble, M. (Ed.), Wiley, 33-48.

Girgis, M. (1986a). Emotional disturbance in limbic system dysfunction. *Int. J. of Neurology*, 19-20: 74-88.

Girgis, M. (1986b). Biochemical patterns in limbic system circuitry: Biochemical-electrophysiological interaction displayed by chemitrode techniques. *The Limbic System, Functional Organization and Clinical Disorders*, B.K. Doane and K.E. Livingston (Eds.), Raven Press, New York.

Girgis, M. (1992). *The Dementias: Crossroads between Neurology and Psychiatry*, Warren H. Green Inc., St Louis.

Girgis, M. and Indik, J. (1986). Limbic epilepsy and the interface with psychiatry. *Biological Psychiatry*. Shagas et al. (Ed.)

Girgis, M. and Kiloh, L. (Eds.). (1980). *Limbic Epilepsy and the Dyscontrol Syndrome*, Elsevier, N. Holland, Amst.

Glaser, G.H. (1967). Limbic epilepsy in childhood. *J. Nervous and Mental Disease*, 144: 391-397.

Glaser, G.H. and Dixon, M.S. (1956). Psychomotor seizures in childhood. *Neurol.*, 6: 646-655.

Gloor, P. (1960). The amygdala. *Handbook of Physiology*, Vol. II, Sec. 1, 1395, Field, Magoun and Hall (Eds.), Am. Phys. Soc., Washington, D.C.

Gloor, P. and Feindel, W. (1963). Temporal lobe and affective behavior. *Physiologie des Vegetativen Nerven Systems*, Vol. II. M. Mannier (Ed.), Stuttgart Hipokrates Verlag.

Goddard, G.V. (1964). Junctions of the amygdala. *Psychol. Bull.*, 62: 89-109.

Goddard, G.V. (1969). Analysis of avoidance conditioning following cholinergic stimulation of amygdala in rats. *J. Comp. Physiol.*, 68 (2). pp. 2: pps. 1-18.

Goddard, G.V. (1980). Kindling model of limbic epilepsy. *Limbic Epilepsy and the Dyscontrol Syndrome*, Girgis, M. & Kiloh, L.G. (Eds.), p. 107-116, Elsevier/North Holland Biomedical Press, Amsterdam.

Goddard, G.V., McIntyre, D.C. and Leech, C.K. (1969). A permanent change in brain function resulting from daily electrical stimulation. *Exp. Neurol.*, 25: 295-330.

Hamilton, M.A. (1967). Development of a rating scale for primary depressive illness, *Br. J. Soc. Clin. Psyoch.*, 6: 27896.

Hammett, V.B.O. (1962). The psychiatrist and psychosomatic medicine. *Psychosomatic Medicine*, Chpt. 119, J.C. Nodine and J.H. Moyer (Eds), Lea & Febiger, Philadelphia: 950-953.

Hancock, J.R. and Walker, C.E. (1990). Adolescence. *Behavior and Medicine*, Danny Wedding (Ed.), Mosby, St Louis.

Himwich, H.E. (1965). *The Scientific Basis of Drug Therapy in Psychiatry*, Marks and Pare (Eds.), Pergamon Press.

Hofstatter, L. and Girgis, M. (1973). Depth Electrode Investigations of the Limbic System with Radio Stimulation, Electrolytic Lesions and Histochemical Techniques. *Surgical Approaches in Psychiatry*, L.V. Laitinen and K.K. Livingston (Eds.), University Park Press, Baltimore.

Hofstatter, L. and Girgis, M. (1979). Neurotransmitter Mechanisms Underlying Psychiatric Surgery, Electroconvulsive Therapy and Antidepressive Drug Therapy. *Modern Concepts in Psychiatric Surgery*, Hitchcock et al. (Ed.), Elsevier North/ Holland, Amsterdam. pp. 2-15.

Hordern, A. (1974). Depressive Disorders. *Practitioner*, 213: 560.

Hornykiewicz, O. (1963). Die Topische Lokalisation und das Vernalten von Noradrenalin und Dopamin (3-hydroxytyramin). *Der Substantia Nigra des Normalen und Parkinson-kranken Mensche*, Wein. Klin. Wochensch, 75: 309-312.

Jackson, J.H. (1899). On asphyxia in slight epileptic paroxysms on the symptomatology of slight epileptic fits supposed to depend on discharge-lesions of the uncinate gyrus. Lancet.

Jackson, H.J. and Stewart, P. (1899). Epileptic attacks with a warning of a crude sensation of smell and with the intellectual aura (dreamy state) in a patient who had symptoms pointing to gross organic disease of the right temporosphenoidal lobe. *Brain*, 22: 534-549.

Janowsky, D.S., El-Yousef, M.K., Davies, J.M. and Sekerks, H.J. (1972). *A Cholinergic-adrenergic Hypotheses of Mania and Depression*, Lancet. 1: 632-634.

Jasper, H.H., Gloor, P. and Milner, B. (1956). *Ann. Rev. Physiol.*, 18: 359.

Kaplan, H.I. and Sadock, B.J. (1989). *Comprehensive Textbook of Psychiatry*, V. Williams and Wilkins.

Katzman, R. (1976). The prevalence and malignancy of Alzheimer's disease: a major killer (Editorial). *Arch. Neurol.*, 33: 217-218.

Katzman, R. (1977). Normal pressure hydrocephalus. *Dementia*, 2nd ed., Hills, C.E. (Ed.), F.A. Davis, Philadelphia.

Kiloh, L.G. (1981). Pseudodementia. *The Crisis of the Aging Mind*, R. Chynoweth and D. Bochner (Eds.), S. Aust. Postgrad. Med. Ed. Assoc. Inc.

Kluver, H. and Bucy, P.C. (1937). "Psychic blindness" and other symptoms following temporal lobectomy in rhesus monkeys. *Amer. J. Physiol.*, 119: 352-353.

Kluver, H. and Bucy, P.C. (1939). Preliminary analysis of functions of the temporal lobes in monkeys. *Arch. Neurol. and Psychiat.*, 42: 979.

Kramer, P. (1993). *Listening to Prozac*, Viking.

Lebensohn, Z.M. and Jenkins, R.B. (1975). Improvement of Parkinsonism in Depressed Patients Treated with ECT. *Amer. J. Psychiat.*, 132: 283-285.

Lehmann, J., Nagy, J.I., Atmadja, S. and Fibigher, H.C. (1980). The nucleus basalis magnocellularis: the origin of a cholinergic projection to the neocortex of the rat. *Neuroscience*, 5: 1161-1174.

Lennox, W.G. (1960). *Epilepsy and Related Disorders*, Little Brown, Boston.

Lorente De No, R. (1938). Analysis of the activity of the chains of the internuntial neurons, *J. Neurophysiol.*, 1:207.

MacLean, P.D. (1949). Psychosomatic disease and the "visceral brain". Recent developments bearing on the Papez theory of emotion. *Psychosom. Med.*, Vol. II, 338-353.

MacLean, P.D. (1958a). Contrasting functions of limbic and neocortical systems and their relevance to psychophysiological aspects of medicine. *Amer. J. Med.*, 25: 611-626.

MacLean, P.D. (1958b). The limbic system with respect to selfpreservation and the preservation in the species. *J. Nerv. Ment. Dis.*, 127: 1-11.

MacLean, P.D. (1970). The limbic brain in relation to psychosis. *Physiological Correlates of Emotion*, Chap. 7, Acad. Press.

MacLean, P.D. and Delgado, J.M.R. (1953). Electrical and chemical stimulation of frontotemporal portion of limbic system in the waking animal. *Electroenceph. Clin. Neurophysiol.*, 5: 91-1 00.

Magnus, O., Penfield, W. and Jasper, H. (1952). Mastication and consciousness in epileptic seizures, *Acta Psychiat. et Neurol.*, 27: 91-115.

Malamud, N. (1967). Psychiatric disorder with intracranial tumors of limbic system. *Arch. Neurol.*, 17: 113-123 .

Mark, V.H. and Ervin, F.R. (1978). *Violence and the Brain*, Harper and Row, New York, pp. 170.

McGeer, E.G., McGeer, P.L. and Singh, K. (1978). Kainic acid induced degeneration of neostriatal neurones: Dependency upon corticostriatal tract. *Brain Res.*, 139: 381-383.

McNamara, J.O. (1978). Muscarinic cholinergic receptors participate in the kindling model of epilepsy. *Brain Res.*, 154: 415.

Meares, A. (1967). *Relief Without Drugs*, Fontana/Collins.

Mellville, J. (1984). *The Tranquillizer Trap*, Fontana/Collins.

Nielsen, Bjarne M. (1993). A comparison of Fluoxetin and Imimpramine in the treatment of outpatients with depression. *Acta Psych.,* Scand.

Olds, J. (1958). Self-stimulation experiments and differentiated reward systems. *Reticular Formation of the Brain,* H.H. Jasper et al. (Eds.), Little, Brown & Co., Boston, 671-687.

Olney, J.W. (1974). Toxic effects of glutamate and related amino acids on the developing central nervous system. *Heritable Disorders of Amino Acid Metabolism,* W.L. Nyhan, John Wiley and Sons (Eds.), New York.

Olney, J.W. (1978). Neurotoxicity of excitatory amino acids. *Kainic Acid as a Tool in Neurobiology,* E.G. McGeer, J.W. Olney and P.L. McGeer (Eds.), Raven Press, New York.

Olney, J.W. and De Gubareff (1978). Glutamate neurotoxicity and Huntington's chorea. *Nature,* 271: 557-559.

Olney, J.W. and Fuller, T.A. (1981). Kainic acid and other excitotoxins: A comparative analysis. *Glutamate as a Neurotransmitter.* G. Chiara and G.L. Gessa (Eds.), Raven Press, New York.

Olney, J.W., Rhee, V. and Ho, O.L. (1974). Kainic Acid: A powerful neurotoxic analogue of glutamate, *Brain Res.,* 77: 507-512.

Olney, J.W., Sharpe, L.G. and De Gubareff, T.S. (1975). Excitotoxic amino acids; *Neurosci. Abstr.,* 1: 371.

Ounstead, C., Lindsay, J. and Norman, R. (1966). Biological factors in temporal lobe epilepsy. *Clinics in Development Medicine,* No. 22, Heineman, London.

Papez, J.W. (1937). A proposed mechanism of emotion. *Arch. Neurol. Psychiat.,* 38: 725-743.

Pastuszac, A. (1993). Pregnancy outcome following first trimester exposure to Fluoxetine (Prozac). *JAMA,* 269:17.

Penfield, W. and Jasper, H. (1954). *Epilepsy and the Functional Anatomy of the Human Brain,* Little, Brown and Co., Boston.

Penfield, W. (1956). Epileptogenic lesions. *Acta Neurol. Psychiat. Belg.,* 5: 75-88.

Perry, E.K., Perry, R.H., Blessed, G. and Tomlinson, B.E. (1977). Necropsy evidence of central cholinergic deficits in senile dementia (Letter). Lancet, 1: 189.

Post, R.M., Pulman, F.W., Ballinger, J.C., Berritlini, W.H. (1982). Kindling and Carbamezepine in affective illness. *J. Nerv., Ment. Dis.,* 170: 717.

Potter, D.D., Furshpan, A.J. and Landis, S.C. (1981). Multiple transmitter status and "Dales Principle". *Neuroscience Commentaries,* Vol. 1: 10-15.

Pribram, K.H. and Kruger, L. (1954). Functions of the "olfactory brain". *Ann. N.Y. Acad. Sci.*, 58: 109-138.

Racine, R. (1972). Modification of seizure activity by electrical simulation: I After-discharge threshold. *Electroenceph. Clin. Neurophysiol.*, 32: 269-279.

Reisine, T.D., Yamamurra, H.I., Bird, E.D., Spokes, E. and Enna, S.T. (1978). Pre and post-synaptic neurochemical alterations in Alzheimer's disease. *Brain Res.*, 159: 477.

Roth, M., Tomlinson, B.E. and Blessed, G. (1966). Correlation between score for dementia and counts of "senile plaques" in cerebral gray matter of elderly subjects. *Nature*, 209: 109.

Rubenstein, L.Z. (1982). Reversible Dementia. *Annals of Int. Med.*, 97.

Seligman, M.E.P. (1975). *Helplessness*, Freeman, San Francisco.

Seligman, M.E.P. (1993). *Learned Optimism*, Random House.

Shute, C.C.D. (1975). Chemical transmitter systems in the brain. *Modern Trends in Neurology*, 6: 183-203.

Snyder, S.H. (1980). Brain peptides and neurotransmitters. *Science*, 209: 976-983.

Spehlman, R., Daniels, J.C. and Chang, C.M. The effects of eserine and atropine on the epileptiform activity of chronically isolated cortex. *Epilepsia*, 12: 123-133.

Sperry, R.W. (1963.) Chemoaffinity in the orderly growth of nerve fiber patters and connections. *Proc. Nat. Acad. Sci. USA*, 50: 703.

Stark, P., Fuller, R.W., Wong, D.T. (1985). The pharmacologic profile of fluoxetine. *J. Clin. Psychiatry*, 46: 7-13.

Stokes, P. (1993). Fluoxetine: A five year review. *Clinical Therapeutic*, 13: 2.

Strang, R.R. (1965). Imipramine in treatment of Parkinsonism: A blind placebo study. *Brit. Med. J.*, 2: 33-34.

Tremblay, E., Ottersen, O.P., Rovira, C. and Ben-Ari, Y. (1983). Intra-amygdaloid injections of kainic acid: regional metabolic changes and their relation to the pathological alterations. *Neuroscience*, Vol. 8, No. 2: 299-314.

Trimble, M.R. (1985). *The Psychopharmacology of Epilepsy*, Wiley.

Ulett, G.A. and Johnson, N.W. (1957). Effect of Atropine and Scopolamine upon electroencephalographic changes induced by electroconvulsive therapy. *EEG Clin. Neurophysiol.*, 9: 217.

Ungar, G. (1970). Molecular mechanisms in information processing. *Int. Rev. Neurobiol.*, 13: 223.

Vosu, H. and Wise, R.A. Cholingergic seizure kindling in the rat: comparison of caudate, amygdala, and hippocampus. *Behav. Biol.*, 12: 491-495.

Votava, Z., Benesova, O., Bohdanecky, Z. and Grofova, O. (1968). Influence of Atropine, Scopolamine and Benactyzine on the Physostigmine Arousal Reaction in Rabbits. *Progress in Brain Research*, P.B. Bradley and M. Fink, Elsevier Publishing Co. (Eds.), New York, pp. 40-47.

Wada, J.A. (1980). Amygdaloid and frontal cortical kindling in subhuman primates. *Limbic Epilepsy and the Dyscontrol Syndrome*, Girgis, M. and Kiloh, L.G. (Eds.), Elsevier/North Holland Amsterdam, pp 120-133.

Wada, J.A. and Sato, M. (1974). Generalized convulsive seizures induced by daily electrical stimulation of the amygdala in cats: correlative, electrographic and behavioural features. *Neurology*, 24: 565-574.

Ward, A. (1950). Atropine in the treatment of closed head injury. *J. Neurosurg.*, 7: 398-402.

Wasterlain, C.G., Holm, S.H. and Jonec, V. (1978). The kindling phenomenon. *Neurology*, 28: 346-347.

Wedding, D. (1990). *Behavior and Medicine*, Mosby, St. Louis.

Wender, P.H. and Kline, D.F. (1981). *Mind, Mood and Medicine*, Farrar, Straus and Giroux, New York.

Wilkinson, S. (1989). *Depression*, London, BMA.

Woert, M.H., Van Ambani, L. and Bowers, M. B. (1972). Levodopa and Cholinergic Hypersensitivity in Parkinson's Disease. *Neurol. Suppl.*, pp. 86-93.

Wofsley, A.R., Kuhar, M.J. and Snyder, S.H. (1971). A unique synaptosomal fraction which accumulates glutamic and aspartic acids in brain tissue. *Proc. Natl. Acad. Sci.*, 68: 1102.

World Health Organization. (1973). Report of the International Pilot Study of Schizophrenia (WHO Geneva, 73).

INDEX